D0146946

Understanding Learning Disability and Dementia

of related interest

Ethical Issues in Dementia Care
Making Difficult Decisions
Julian C. Hughes and Clive Baldwin
ISBN 978 1 84310 357 8

Person-Centred Dementia Care
Making Services Better
Dawn Brooker
ISBN 978 1 84310 337 0

Design for Nature in Dementia Care
Garuth Chalfont
ISBN 978 1 84310 571 8

Involving Families in Care Homes
A Relationship-Centred Approach to Dementia Care
Bob Woods, John Keady and Diane Seddon
ISBN 978 1 84310 229 8

Healing Arts Therapies and Person-Centred Dementia Care
Edited by Anthea Innes and Karen Hatfield
ISBN 978 1 84310 038 6

Primary Care and Dementia
Steve Iliffe and Vari Drennan
Foreword by Murna Downs
ISBN 978 1 85302 997 4

Advance Directives in Mental Health
Theory, Practice and Ethics
Jacqueline Atkinson
ISBN 978 1 84310 483 4

Ageing, Disability and Spirituality
Addressing the Challenge of Disability in Later Life
Edited by Elizabeth MacKinlay
ISBN 978 184310 584 8

RC
521
.K47
2007

Understanding Learning Disability and Dementia

Developing Effective Interventions

Diana Kerr

17111889

NYACK COLLEGE MANHATTAN

Jessica Kingsley Publishers
London and Philadelphia

First published in 2007
by Jessica Kingsley Publishers
116 Pentonville Road
London N1 9JB, UK
and
400 Market Street, Suite 400
Philadelphia, PA 19106, USA

www.jkp.com

Copyright © Diana Kerr 2007

All rights reserved. No part of this publication may be reproduced in any material form (including photocopying or storing it in any medium by electronic means and whether or not transiently or incidentally to some other use of this publication) without the written permission of the copyright owner except in accordance with the provisions of the Copyright, Designs and Patents Act 1988 or under the terms of a licence issued by the Copyright Licensing Agency Ltd, Saffron House, 6-10 Kirby Street, London EC1N 8TS. Applications for the copyright owner's written permission to reproduce any part of this publication should be addressed to the publisher.

Warning: The doing of an unauthorised act in relation to a copyright work may result in both a civil claim for damages and criminal prosecution.

Library of Congress Cataloging in Publication Data
A CIP catalog record for this book is available from the Library of Congress

British Library Cataloguing in Publication Data
A CIP catalogue record for this book is available from the British Library

ISBN 978 1 84310 442 1

Printed and bound in Great Britain by
Athenaeum Press, Gateshead, Tyne and Wear

Contents

Acknowledgements

An enormous amount of thanks goes to Brian Kerr for reading the manuscript so diligently and for giving important advice and critical comment. Also he has my admiration for bearing with the endless moans and groans that accompanied the writing of this book.

Thanks go to Colm Cunningham, who persuaded me to write this book. Also thanks for his forbearance in the face of endless threats to quit the whole enterprise.

Chris Lawes' admirable attention to grammatical detail was sorely tested and proved invaluable. Thank you.

I also wish to thank the Trustees of the Dementia Services Development Centre at the University of Stirling and the H.E. Mitchell's Charitable Trust for their support in the production of this book.

The author would like to thank the publishers and authors who have kindly given permission to reproduce the following material:

Buijssen, H. (2005) *The Simplicity of Dementia*. London: Jessica Kingsley Publishers, Copyright © Huub Buijssen.

Cairns, D. and Kerr, D. (1994) *Different Realities: A Training Guide for People with Down's Syndrome and Alzheimer's Disease*. Stirling: Dementia Services Development Centre, University of Stirling, Copyright © The Dementia Services Development Centre.

Dodd, K., Kerr, D. and Fern, S. (2006) *Down's Syndrome and Dementia: Workbook for Staff*. Teddington: Down's Syndrome Association, Copyright © Down's Syndrome Association.

Earnshaw, K. and Donnelly, V. (2001) 'The differential diagnosis chart', in 'Partnerships in practice.' *Learning Disability Practice 4*, 3, 27.

Kerr, D., Cunningham, C. and Wilkinson, H. (2006) *Responding to the Pain Needs of People with a Learning Disability and Dementia*. York: York Publishing Services, Copyright © Joseph Rowntree Foundation. Reproduced by permission of the Joseph Rowntree Foundation.

Murphy, C. (1994) *'It started with a Sea-shell': Life Story Work and People with Dementia.* Stirling: Dementia Services Development Centre, University of Stirling, Copyright © The Dementia Services Development Centre.

Pollock, A. (2001) *Designing Gardens for People with Dementia.* Stirling: Dementia Service Development Centre, University of Stirling, © The Dementia Services Development Centre.

VOICES (Voluntary Organisations Involved in Caring in the Elderly Sector) (1998) *Eating Well for Older People with Dementia: A Good Practice Guide for Residential and Nursing Homes and Others Involved in Caring for Older People with Dementia: Report of an Expert Working Group.* Potters Bar: VOICES and Gardner Merchant Healthcare Services. The materials are available via the Caroline Walker Trust website, www.cwt.org.uk (accessed 9 May 2007) and reproduced by permission of the Association of Charity Officers.

Introduction

People with learning disability, along with the rest of the population, are living longer. This increased longevity brings with it the conditions and illnesses of older age. Dementia is one of these conditions. Whilst there is no agreement on the extent of the condition amongst people with a learning disability from causes other than Down's syndrome, it is probably correct to say that they do have a slightly higher prevalence rate of dementia than the general population (Janicki and Dalton 2000). People with Down's syndrome, however, have a significantly higher prevalence rate than the general population (Prasher 2005). Those people who do develop the condition also tend to have an earlier age of onset than the general population (Prasher 2005).

Case study 1

Alistair is 52 years old and has Down's syndrome. He has been living in a supported house for the past eight years after coming out of a long-stay hospital where he had lived since he was 5 years old.

Over the past eight years Alistair has developed many new skills. He has attended college courses, developed a close relationship with Jennifer, whom he met at college, and has increasingly taken responsibility for his own daily routines. He shares his house with three other men, two of whom were in the hospital with him.

Over the last nine months Alistair has started to change. He has lost some of his of daily living skills. He puts clothes on in the wrong order, often putting two or more jumpers on at once. Doing up his shoes has become an almost impossible task. He needs prompting to shave both sides of his face and will become very agitated in the bathroom. He will sit and stare at his food, in stark contrast to his previous approach to food, which was to eat at breakneck speed.

He has, on a number of occasions, been found 'wandering' around the streets after he returns from his day service on the bus. He has twice gone into the wrong house in the terrace in which he lives. Alistair has also become quite agitated and is quick to shout and on one occasion, quite uncharacteristically, hit out at a member of staff at his day service.

The day service provider is questioning whether Alistair can continue to attend. Staff at his house are concerned that he needs more support than is, at present, available.

Alistair may have dementia. He needs a proper diagnosis and the provision of appropriate and responsive resources so that he can be supported to maintain skills as long as possible, reduce his anxiety and remain surrounded by familiar friends, carers and environments.

If people with a learning disability who develop dementia are to receive the quality and level of care and support they need, it is essential that care commissioners, commissioners of services, providers, support staff, family, informal carers and indeed regulators know more about the condition, its impact on people with a learning disability, their care needs and the components that need to be in place for the provision of appropriate, coherent and consistent models of care and policies. This book will address all these issues.

People with a learning disability who develop dementia do not always remain within the learning disability service. Sometimes they are supported and cared for within older people's services. This means that two distinct groups of staff and service providers may often be involved in their care. These two groups will have different expertise as well as different areas of weakness. Many staff, professionals and organisations will have plenty of experience of supporting people with a learning disability but know little about dementia. Many individuals who work with people with a learning disability will have much experience and training on issues related to younger people but not so much in relation to issues that are pertinent to older people with a learning disability (Kerr, Cunningham and Wilkinson 2006). Others will have experience of working with older people with dementia but little experience of people with a learning disability (Kerr 1997). This book should be useful for all these groups of staff.

Understanding Learning Disability and Dementia is a book about practice with an emphasis on the use of psychosocial interventions. Case study material has been used throughout to help to illustrate issues and to enable the reader to identify with the problems and challenges that these examples present. The book can be read sequentially but it is also anticipated that readers will dip into it and use the various chapters as stand-alone guides to specific practice issues.

Chapter 1 provides a brief account of what constitutes a learning disability. Some examples are given of some of the more common causes. The chapter is not intended to be comprehensive but is intended for people whose work and personal life have provided little or no experience of people with a learning disability.

Chapter 2 describes the most common dementias and their prevalence rates amongst people with a learning disability. The chapter provides a basic introduction to the brain and its functions. It is not necessary to have a detailed knowledge of the brain to understand the person with dementia. However, some idea about the distribution of functions should help to explain some of the changes that occur. There is also a list of the important early signs of the onset of the condition.

Chapter 3 tackles the complex and often fraught issue of getting a diagnosis. The chapter provides information about the various conditions that can be confused with dementia. It also provides a tool to enable staff to identify possible causes of changes in a person's behaviour that may look like but are not caused by dementia. The chapter looks at reasons for delay in referral for assessment and diagnosis and offers some solutions.

Chapter 4 addresses the fact that people with dementia will increasingly believe themselves to be living in the past. They will often have a different reality from people without dementia. The chapter gives examples to help the reader better understand the world from the perspective of the person with dementia. It also describes and evaluates the different responses that can be used.

Chapter 5 focuses on communication. People with learning disabilities may already have problems with communication, which are exacerbated when they develop dementia. The chapter argues for an increased awareness and use of non-verbal forms of communication such as touch and music. It provides information on what to avoid and what to use to enhance and facilitate good verbal communication.

Chapter 6 describes and evaluates a number of therapeutic interventions such as the use of failure-free activities, reminiscence work, life story work, touch, music and aromatherapy. These can not only help to minimise distress, loss of self-esteem, and anxiety but also help to maintain skills and involvement with others.

Chapter 7 focuses on the understanding, prevention and management of 'challenging behaviour'. The chapter emphasises the fact that carers and the physical environment induce most challenging behaviours in people with dementia. This means that there is much that carers and service providers can do to prevent challenging behaviour. The chapter explains some ways in which this behaviour can be triggered and the potential use of ABC charts in the understanding and analysis of the behaviour. The issues of what is often referred to pejoratively as 'wandering' and night-time disturbance are given particular attention.

Chapter 8 describes the experiences and management of pain amongst people with a learning disability and dementia. The chapter suggests many reasons why this experience is not managed well and provides information on ways in which practice can be improved.

Chapter 9 considers the experiences and needs of the peers of people with a learning disability and dementia. It gives information on useful materials to help them understand what is happening to the person with dementia. These materials should also enable them to raise any fears they may have about their own vulnerability to the condition. There is discussion about the fact that the acknowledgement that someone has dementia does raise issues of confidentiality and disclosure that need to be addressed.

Chapter 10 identifies the problems with eating and drinking that people with dementia are likely to develop. The social, emotional and physical aspects of the problems are identified and a number of solutions are suggested. The use of percutaneous endoscopic gastrosomy (PEG) is described and considered.

Chapter 11 focuses on the issue of the physical environment and its impact on people with a learning disability and dementia. The chapter highlights the way in which the environment can disable people with a learning disability and dementia and offers examples of how design and adaptations to the environment can enable and support people with dementia.

Chapter 12 describes how the increasing number of technologies that are being developed can enable the person with dementia to be safer and potentially have an improved quality of life.

Chapter 13 addresses the issues around end stage care. The need to engage input from specialist professionals is emphasised. The changes that are likely to be experienced by the person with a learning disability and dementia are given along with guidelines and advice for staff and carers on how best to respond and support the person at the end stage.

Chapter 14 is about the concerns and needs of relatives. Staff need to be sensitive to the needs of families, and to engage them proactively in care for and decisions about the family member with dementia. Staff also need to be aware of the feelings of guilt and failure that can sometimes underlie complaints about the level of care that the person with dementia is being given.

Chapter 15 is about medication. It provides information about the impact of some medication on people with dementia and in particular on the use of antipsychotic medication. The role and impact of cholinesterase inhibitors in the early stages of the condition is also discussed.

Chapter 16 is about models of care. It describes and considers the pros and cons of three models of provision, 'ageing in place', 'in place progression' and 'referral out'. It also briefly describes a fourth model, 'outreach'.

The book concludes with a personal plea for the future.

What is a Learning Disability?

In this book the term 'learning disability' will be used to describe the group of people who are its subjects. However, it should be noted that both nationally and internationally there is not one agreed term to describe this grouping. People in the UK use terms such as 'learning disability' or 'learning difficulty' and previously used the term 'mentally handicapped'. In the USA the term 'mental retardation' has been used until very recently. A newer term of 'intellectual disability' is gaining popularity in both North America and Europe. Most people, however, recognise the need for an appropriate and meaningful description of people who may need specialised services or other support because of a significant intellectual deficit or disability.

It is not within the remit of this book to catalogue the various syndromes and types of learning disability. This chapter provides some basic information to people who do not generally work with people with a learning disability.

The group of people being described under the term 'learning disability' will have a significant lifelong condition, which has three facets:

- reduced ability to understand new or complex information or to use new skills

- reduced ability to cope independently

- a condition that started before adulthood (before the age of 18 years) with a lasting effect on the individual's development (Scottish Executive 2000).

Sometimes the severity of the person's learning disability is also recorded in terms of IQ (intelligent quotient). The broad categories are as follows:

- mild learning disability   IQ 70–50
- moderate learning disability   IQ 50–35
- severe learning disability   IQ 35–20
- profound learning disability   IQ less than 20.

About 66 per cent of the general population have an IQ of 85–115. About 1.5 million people in the UK have a learning disability of some sort. Every week 200 babies are born with a learning disability (Mencap 2006).

The number of people with a learning disability is expanding. In the 35-year period from 1960 to 1995 there was a 53 per cent increase that represented an annual increase of 1.2 per cent (McGrother *et al.* 2001). This increase is substantially the result of improvements in socio-economic conditions and improvements in neonatal care resulting in improved survival rates. A further increase between 1995 and 2008 of 11 per cent is predicted, the consequence of increased longevity of people with a learning disability (McGrother *et al.* 2001). People with a learning disability from causes other than Down's syndrome would be expected to have a similar life span to members of the general population. People with Down's syndrome would have a shorter expectancy but still often live into their late sixties and early seventies. It is also important to note that increased survival rates and subsequent longevity has led to an increase in people at all ages with severe levels of disability.

The term 'learning disability' covers a wide range of conditions. These have highly varied presentations and widely different consequences for the people who have them. The impact of the learning disability on people will be highly varied. No two people will experience their disability in the same way. People with a learning disability are individuals with highly varied abilities and personalities. Like people without a disability they are the product of their life experience, history and cultural expectations as well as their genetic inheritance.

People with a learning disability will often have difficulty with communication; but they do want to communicate. They will often look different in some way; this can be unnerving for some people. It is important to look beyond the physical differences and see the person that is there. What is important is that, no matter what the disability, the person has the same needs and rights as a non-disabled person.

There are many different causes of learning disability. Events before, during and after birth can all be responsible.

- Before birth
  - damage to the central nervous system
  - mother has an illness or a physical accident during pregnancy
  - genetic inheritance
- During birth
  - insufficient oxygen during the birth or premature birth
- After birth
  - early childhood illnesses or physical accidents.

Inherited causes of learning disability

The most common inherited causes of learning disability are Fragile X syndrome and Down's syndrome. Because people with Down's syndrome will have a higher prevalence of dementia than people with any other type of learning disability and it is the most common cause of developmental delay, intellectual impairment and learning disability, more attention has been given to this condition.

Down's syndrome

- Two babies with Down's syndrome are born every day in the UK. Around one in every thousand babies born will have Down's syndrome.
- There are 60,000 people in the UK with the condition.
- Although the individual chance of a baby having Down's syndrome is higher for older mothers, more babies with Down's syndrome are born to younger women, reflecting the higher birth rate in this group.
- Down's syndrome is caused by the presence of an extra chromosome in a baby's cells. It occurs by chance at conception and is irreversible.

- Down's syndrome is not a disease. People with Down's syndrome are not ill and do not 'suffer' from the condition.

Down's syndrome results from the inheritance of a third copy of all or part of chromosome 21. People without Down's syndrome have two copies of chromosome 21. There are three types of Down's syndrome: Trisomy 21, Mosaic Down's syndrome and Translocation Down's syndrome.

Trisomy 21 is the most common form of the syndrome. It occurs just before or at the point of conception. It happens when chromosome 21 in either the sperm or the egg does not separate properly and then the chromosome is duplicated in every cell of the body. This means that the person has three rather than two copies of chromosome 21. Of people with Down's syndrome, 95 per cent will have this form of the condition.

Mosaic Down's syndrome occurs after conception. In this case the duplication of chromosome 21 is present only in some cells. The number of cells that have the duplicated chromosome will determine the extent to which the person is affected by the condition.

Translocation Down's syndrome occurs as in Trisomy where there are three chromosomes 21 but in this case one of the chromosomes 21 attaches itself to another chromosome and does not separate. This type of Down's syndrome occurs when one parent carries the gene that is responsible for the condition.

People with Down's syndrome will have a number of physical characteristics. These are given below. Whilst this is interesting as information about the person's physical appearance, it does not tell us anything about the person and it is important that we see beyond these characteristics.

The most common physical characteristics are:

- flat back of head
- abundant neck skin
- flat facial appearance
- slanted eyes
- epicanthic folds (a fold of skin of the upper eyelid that partially covers the inner corner of the eye)
- small teeth
- furrowed tongue

- high arched palate
- short broad hands
- curved fifth finger
- four finger crease on the palm
- wide space between the first and second toe
- speckling of the iris
- congenital heart defects
- gastro-intestinal abnormalities
- muscle hypotonia (decreased muscle tone)
- hyperextensibility or hyperflexibility
- cervical spine instability
- shortness of stature.

Some of these will have added significance when people grow older and also if they develop dementia. This is dealt with later in the book.

People with Down's syndrome will have varying degrees of disability. Some people will be severely disabled and require lots of support and care. Others, perhaps the majority, will experience only minor problems and many, with the right support, will be able to lead fairly independent lives.

The life expectancy of people with Down's syndrome has increased dramatically since the 1950s. In 1929 the average life expectancy was 9 years; by 1949 it had increased to 12 years. Nowadays about 80 per cent of people with Down's syndrome will live to over 50 and many will reach their late sixties and early seventies.

Fragile X syndrome

Fragile X syndrome is a recently discovered disorder. It is thought to affect as many as 5 per cent of people with a learning disability, mainly males. Not all people with Fragile X will have a learning disability. As in Down's syndrome, chromosome 21 is implicated. It is due to a constriction on the long arm of the chromosome in many cells. There is a high degree of variation in the level of disability amongst people with this syndrome. The most common characteristics include social anxiety, avoiding eye contact, poor concentration and speech disorder.

Prader-Willi syndrome

Prader-Willi syndrome occurs in about 1 in 10,000 live births. There is evidence of some chromosomal damage to chromosome 15. Babies have very poor muscle tone. One characteristic of this syndrome is that people often have a need to eat constantly; sometimes this means that they will steal food. They will, as a consequence of their eating, be overweight. They are often also short in stature.

Conditions sometimes associated with a learning disability

There are some conditions that are often associated with a learning disability. However, many people will have one of the conditions listed below but will not have a learning disability.

Autism

Autism is a lifelong disability that affects the way someone communicates and relates to people around them. It is not itself a learning disability, but some people with autism do have a learning disability. It can present as mild, moderate or severe. People with autism may have difficulties in forming relationships with other people, communicating and understanding what other people are trying to communicate, and using their imagination. About 91 in every 10,000 people in the UK have autism (Mencap 2006).

Asperger's syndrome

Asperger's syndrome is a form of autism. Like autism, it is not a learning disability. It can affect the way someone communicates with and relates to other people. People with Asperger's syndrome can find it difficult to tell how other people are feeling by looking at the expression on their faces or listening to the tone of their voices. They usually have fewer problems with language than people with autism. Typically they often like to have a regular routine and can find changes to this upsetting (Mencap 2006). People with Asperger's syndrome are less likely to have a learning disability than people with autism. Indeed they often have average or above average intelligence.

Cerebral palsy

Cerebral palsy is a physical condition which affects people's movement. It can be mild, moderate or severe. Cerebral palsy is not a learning disability, but many people with a learning disability also have cerebral palsy.

Epilepsy

Epilepsy is not a learning disability, but about 30 per cent of people with a learning disability also have epilepsy. People with epilepsy have seizures. A seizure happens when there is a problem with activity in the brain.

Changing attitudes and practice

Policy and practice since the mid-1980s have increasingly focused on the need to move away from the institutionalising and often dehumanising experiences of people with a learning disability. The work of Wolfensberger (1972) and O'Brien (1987) highlighted the need to change attitudes and practice towards people with a learning disability. This led to a movement in the UK to support people with a learning disability to have meaningful lives, experiences and opportunities, to enable them to reach their true potential and engage as far as possible in the lives of the communities in which they lived. The move from normalisation, through social role valorisation, inclusion and person-centred planning has been a long journey that has enriched many lives and resulted in a significant cultural shift in the way in which people with a learning disability are perceived and responded to.

It is imperative that these advances are not lost when people get older and/or develop dementia. There is a need to make certain that learning disability services do not adopt the ageist attitudes and practices that often characterise older people's services. Further it is vital that staff who work within the older people's services are able to maintain and replicate the attitudes and practices that have been developed and embedded within the learning disability service. The work of Thompson and Wright (2001) and Wilkinson *et al.* (2004) suggests that there is a need for vigilance if people with a learning disability are not going to be discriminated against and suffer the effects of ageism either within the learning disability service or when moved into older people's services.

Summary

About 1.5 million people in the UK have a learning disability. This number is set to increase as people with a learning disability experience the benefits of improvements in socio-economic conditions and health care. The increase in numbers is substantially the result of the increased longevity which people with a learning disability now experience. People with a learning disability, from causes other than Down's syndrome, can expect to have a similar life span to the rest of the population. People with Down's syndrome can expect to live into their late sixties and early seventies. There are many different causes of learning disability and many different conditions and syndromes. No two people will experience their disability in the same way. People's personalities, coping mechanisms, history and support will all have an impact, as will the manifestations of the condition.

Policy and practice since the mid-1980s increasingly focused on the need to move away from the institutionalising and often dehumanising services for people with a learning disability. There has been a move to provide people with meaningful, valued lives and experiences. This has often resulted in dramatic improvements in the quality of the lives of people with a learning disability. It is imperative that these gains are not lost as people move into old age and that older people with a learning disability are not subjected to the consequences of the ageist attitudes and provision that exist for the general population.

2

What is Dementia?

'Dementia' is an umbrella term used to describe a wide variety of diseases and disorders of the brain. It is a 'syndrome' characterised by a decline in cognitive function and memory from previously attained intellectual levels, which is sustained over a period of months or years. The deterioration is of such severity that it impairs the affected individual's ability to work and to perform activities of daily living, including communication (Molloy and Lubiniski 1995). 'Consciousness is not clouded; Impairments of cognitive functions are commonly accompanied and occasionally preceded by deterioration in emotional control, social behaviour and motivation' (World Health Organization (WHO) 1992).

Types of dementia

These definitions are relevant to all dementias, although the type of dementia will affect some of the symptoms and the progression of the condition.

The most frequently experienced dementias are:

- Alzheimer's type dementia
- vascular or multi-infarct dementia
- dementia of Lewy body type
- frontal lobe dementia
- Pick's disease
- Parkinson's disease dementia
- Huntington's disease dementia
- alcohol-related dementia
- AIDS-related dementia.

It is not necessary, for the purposes of this book, to describe all these dementias. The most common will be briefly described.

Alzheimer's type dementia

Alzheimer's type dementia accounts for around 55 per cent of patients diagnosed with dementia (Killeen 2000). It is a degenerative disease affecting the brain. The changes are caused by the production of plaques (which contain a protein called beta-amyloid), and neurofibrillary tangles which form in areas of brain tissue and destroy them (Burns, Howard and Pettit 1997). The cause of this process is not yet fully understood. The temporal and parietal lobes of the brain are generally affected in Alzheimer's type dementia, which can result in significant memory loss and an inability to recognise people and places. This can be extremely distressing, particularly if the person no longer recognises his or her image or that of friends and family (Kitwood 1997).

As the condition progresses, basic skills and capabilities will be lost. Visual-spatial skills can become impaired, resulting in the patient becoming unable to put sequences of an activity or movement together: for example, placing their arm into their clothing (Jenkins 1998). The frontal lobe can also be affected and this can result in difficulties in communication and judgement resulting in disinhibited behaviour (Jacques and Jackson 2000). In Alzheimer's type dementia the symptoms progress gradually but persistently over time (Burns *et al.* 1997).

Vascular dementia

Vascular dementia, also referred to as multi-infarct dementia, is another common type of dementia. It is caused by problems in the circulation of blood to the brain, which results in multiple strokes to brain tissue, leading to significant cognitive impairment (Sander 2002). These strokes can result in damage to areas of the brain responsible for speech or language and can produce generalised symptoms of dementia. As a result, vascular dementia may appear similar to Alzheimer's type dementia.

Vascular dementia can progress in an irregular manner with episodes of sudden loss. It can also take the pattern of gradual change, as in Alzheimer's type dementia. The rate of memory loss and insight associated with vascular dementia appears to progress at a slower rate than in Alzheimer's type dementia.

Vascular dementia has been identified as a distinct condition in up to 20 per cent of people with dementia (Miller and Morris 1993); however, as with all types of dementia it can coexist with other forms of the condition. Vascular dementia is considered the second most common form of dementia in the Western world (Nor, McIntosh and Jackson 2005).

Dementia of the Lewy body type

Another common form of dementia is Lewy body dementia. Lewy bodies are tiny spots containing deposits of a protein called alpha-synuclein. These are found in the hippocampus, temporal lobe and neocortex in addition to the classic sites in the substantia nigra and other subcortical regions (Del Ser *et al.* 2000). Patients with Parkinson's disease also have Lewy bodies, but it is the higher density of these in Lewy body dementia that differentiates between the two conditions (McKeith *et al.* 1995).

Lewy body dementia often results in fluctuations in cognitive impairment, which lead to episodic confusion and lucid intervals. These fluctuations in cognition can occur over minutes, hours or days. They can occur in as many of 50–70 per cent of patients and are associated with shifting levels of attention and alertness (Archibald 2003).

Patients with Lewy body dementia can experience visual and auditory hallucinations, secondary delusions and falls. These symptoms can result in the person presenting with behaviours that are challenging. Treatment plans, therefore, may include consideration of the use of neuroleptic (antipsychotic) medication; however, there needs to be extreme caution in the use of antipsychotic medication. This is because people with Lewy body dementia have neuroleptic sensitivity. One study identified that 50 per cent of patients with Lewy body dementia receiving neuroleptic medication had life-threatening adverse effects, including sedation, immobility, rigidity, postural instability, falls and increased confusion. Dehydration, another feature of this disease, is often associated with poor outcomes such as increased mortality rates (Barber, Panikkar and McKeith 2001); therefore, a greater awareness of this form of dementia is important.

Lewy body dementia is ranked as the third major type of dementia. One estimate is that around 20 per cent of people with dementia will have the Lewy body form of the disease (McKeith *et al.* 1995). Another estimate (Del Ser *et al.* 2000) suggests that the figure may be closer to 36 per cent.

It is important to emphasise, however, that even when people have the same type of dementia they can experience it differently and can present different symptoms, characteristics and behaviours. The impact of the condition on people will be determined by their previous health experiences, their personality, the existence of any other disability, their social and cultural history and their coping mechanisms.

Additionally, although the damage is irreversible it is characteristic of people with dementia to be more receptive some days than others and even to change throughout the course of the day. This may be in part due to an on-off impulse in the transmission of signals in the cells or because the person has fewer resources to call on, so is much more likely to be affected by things like tiredness, stress, anxiety and physical illness.

The brain and its functions

The progression of the condition into different areas of the brain will impair and destroy the function of that part of the brain. It is not essential to have a detailed knowledge of the brain to understand the person with dementia. It can be useful, however, to know how the different functions are grouped. This helps in the understanding of specific behaviours and, more importantly, in the understanding of paradoxical behaviours that often appear. It also helps in making decisions about which skills and behaviours are to be encouraged and maintained and which are lost to function forever. What follows is a basic introduction to the different parts of the brain, their functions and which behaviours they stimulate or control.

Temporal lobes

The temporal lobes are located on either side of the brain (see Figure 2.1). The left or dominant lobe stores verbal memory. The right side lobe stores visual memory. Smell and taste are located on both sides. These lobes are involved in our ability to learn new things. Recent memory is laid, recorded and stored and then moved back and stored deep inside the temporal lobes. With the onset of dementia, damage occurs to the lobes and recent memory is lost. Frequently used and strongly stored memories will remain for some time, but, as the disease progresses, these too will be lost.

Parietal lobes

The parietal lobes are also located on either side of the brain, with each side having a specific function. The left side is the analytical and logical centre and is the area that controls patterning. It is therefore important in our use of language, which involves the patterning of words, in our ability to do arithmetic and hence manage money and in our understanding of the pattern or geography of our body. This lobe tells us which is our right side and which our left, critical information when dressing.

When this lobe is damaged people will have difficulty constructing sentences and with reading and writing. They will also have difficulty with dressing. This is important for carers to know, because once the ability to remember patterns has gone, no amount of explaining or showing will get the patterns back. There will come a point, for example, when the person can no longer dress himself or herself. However, it may be that the person

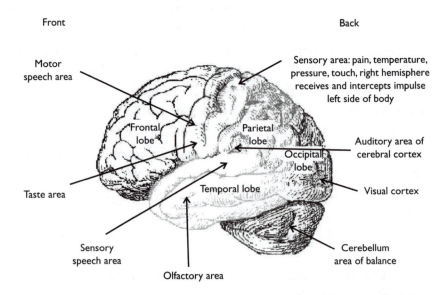

Figure 2.1 Side view of brain. Source: The Dementia Services Development Centre (1997)

can remember two patterns but not three so one needs to be cautious in deciding when all function has gone.

The right side lobe is our three-dimensional centre. This tells us where we are in space and helps us to get around our environment. Once this is damaged people will have difficulty in locating themselves and in making sense of their surroundings. In particular they will have difficulty in seeing changes of levels and will often misinterpret changes in texture and colour, seeing steps where there are none and not seeing those that are there.

Frontal lobes

New learning takes place in the frontal lobes before being passed back into the parietal lobes. This is our planning and organising centre. Importantly, in understanding some behaviour seen in Alzheimer's disease, it is also where our 'initiator' is. This is the part that gets us motivated to do things. When this is damaged people may sit and do nothing, not because they cannot act but because their initiator cannot get them going. If someone else takes the role of initiator, then the person will engage in activity. One problem, however, is that once the person has started to do something, the initiator does not switch off automatically and they may continue to do the same thing over and over again (perseveration) until prompted into doing something else. These lobes are also where we store our knowledge of socially appropriate behaviour.

Limbic region

The limbic region controls sleep, appetite and emotions. It can be disrupted when the frontal and temporal lobes are affected.

Cerebellum

The cerebellum controls balance and the coordination of voluntary movements such as walking and sitting.

Hypothalamus

The hypothalamus works to produce homeostasis, a state of equilibrium. It regulates the body's metabolism. It is the part of the brain that controls hunger, thirst and body temperature. It influences food intake, weight regulation, fluid intake and balance, thirst, body heat and the sleep cycle. The hypothalamus also controls the action of the pituitary gland.

Brain functions

Functions are not necessarily restricted to one area of the brain. This can help to explain why people will sometimes retain some functions even when the primary site for that function is damaged. Those functions that are related to memory, for example, are located in a number of areas.

Dementia and people with a learning disability

There has not been much research into the prevalence and incidence of dementia amongst people who have a learning disability with causes other than Down's syndrome. The research that is available suggests that for people with a learning disability with causes other than Down's syndrome there is a prevalence rate that, whilst not as high as for people with Down's syndrome, is higher than would be found in the general population (Cooper 1997). Three studies (Cooper 1997; Lund 1985; Moss and Patel 1993) found the following prevalence rates of dementia amongst people with a learning disability:

- Aged over 50   13.0 per cent
- Aged over 65   22.0 per cent

A comparison with figures of the prevalence of dementia amongst the general population shows a marked difference.

Prevalence rates amongst the general population:

- Aged 30–59 years   0.1 per cent
- Aged 60–64 years   1.0 per cent
- Aged 65–69 years   1.4 per cent
- Aged 70–74 years   4.1 per cent
- Aged 75–79 years   5.7 per cent
- Aged 80–84 years   13.0 per cent

(Adapted from Hofman *et al.* (1991))

Cooper (1999, p. 129) states that this indicates 'about four times higher [prevalence] than one would expect from an age matched general population'.

Evenhuis (1997) reports that in relation to one dementia, Alzheimer's disease, people with a learning disability from causes other than Down's syndrome are generally at no greater risk than the general population. She suggests that, for these people, Alzheimer's type dementia will occur around 65–75 years. What these various figures do not reveal, because they cover all learning disabilities other than Down's syndrome, is if there are particular syndromes and causes of learning disability that may increase a predisposition for dementia. It may also be the case that some causes of learning disability, particularly single gene disorders, may act as a protection against some dementias (Wherrett 1998).

The reasons for a generally increased risk within the learning disabled population of developing dementia are not clearly known. There are a number of circumstances and peculiarities amongst the population that might explain this increased susceptibility. People with a learning disability may be at increased risk because of acquired brain injury associated with traumatic brain damage (Breteler *et al.* 1992), infection and nutritional deficiency (Janicki and Dalton 1998). Seizures that commonly accompany learning disability may induce changes to the brain that increase the possibility of cognitive impairment (Lynch, Rutecki and Sutula 1996). There is also evidence that low levels of education may predispose people to the onset of Alzheimer's type dementia (Katzman 1993).

The dearth of research around learning disability and dementia amongst people without Down's syndrome is not replicated amongst people with Down's syndrome. There has been a concentration on this group. This is substantially because there is known to be a link between the two conditions and also because the baby boomers, born shortly after the Second World War, are now reaching their fifties and sixties, when they are at increased risk of developing the condition. Amongst people with a learning disability from causes other than Down's syndrome, they will probably not develop the condition at such an early age and so the baby boomers in this population are not yet presenting with dementia in such high numbers. For people with Down's syndrome there is a clear increased susceptibility to the early onset of Alzheimer's type dementia. Studies vary slightly but the following figures are the findings from one study (Prasher 1995) and show the prevalence rate of Alzheimer's type dementia amongst people with Down's syndrome.

- Aged 30–39 years   2 per cent
- Aged 40–49 years   9.4 per cent
- Aged 50–59 years   36.1 per cent
- Aged 60–69 years   54.5 per cent

Different studies have found different mean ages of onset of the condition: these have suggested variations between 51.7 years (Prasher and Krishnan 1993) and Lai and Williams (1989) finding of 54.2 years. Interestingly Prasher and Krishnan (1993) found a difference between the mean age of onset amongst men and women. Men had a mean age of onset of 54.2 years whilst women had 49.8 years. It appears that there is an age-related risk of dementia similar to the general population but between 30 and 40 years earlier.

These figures show that people with Down's syndrome have a much higher rate of Alzheimer's type dementia than the general population. What they also show, however, is that not everyone with Down's syndrome develops the condition. The most favoured explanation of the link between Down's syndrome and dementia is the existence of the third chromosome 21 (people without Down's syndrome have two chromosome 21).

This chromosome is involved in the production of the beta-amyloid protein, which is found in the knots and tangles in the brains of people with Alzheimer's dementia. Almost everyone with Down's syndrome will have these knots and tangles deposited on their brain by the time they are 40. What is important to note, however, is that few of them will, at this stage, have the clinical symptoms of dementia and indeed some may never develop the symptoms. No one has yet been able to explain this fully.

Research by Holland *et al.* (2000) indicates that many people with Down's syndrome may experience frontal lobe changes that predate the onset of the Alzheimer's disease. The characteristics of this stage are often:

- impaired performance on executive function tasks
- preserved episodic memory
- changes in mood, motivation, and stereotypic and challenging behaviour.

It can be difficult to determine the early changes that occur as a result of the dementia. Many of the indicators of dementia are an exaggeration of already existing behaviours and deficits that exist because of the person's learning disability. The early signs of dementia amongst people with a learning disability may well be a further deterioration of an already present deficit, whereas in the general population the loss will be from an area of full competence, and so more easily recognised. There will also be new losses in areas in which the person with a learning disability may well have had full competency.

The following are the early signs that should alert carers to the possibility of the onset of dementia amongst people with a learning disability:

- deterioration in the ability to accomplish skills of daily living
- deterioration in short-term memory
- increased apathy and increased inactivity
- loss of amenability and sociability
- loss of interest in favoured hobbies
- withdrawal of spontaneous communication
- reduction in communication skills
- disorientation and confusion
- changes in depth perception
- changes in night-time sleep patterns
- increased problems with comprehension
- increased wandering.

It is important to emphasise that these difficulties and behaviours are changes from the person's normal behaviour. If someone exhibits three or more of the above changes then a referral should be made for an assessment to determine if these changes are an indication of dementia. The possibility that they are the result of other conditions needs to be eliminated through the application of a differential diagnosis. This is discussed further in Chapter 3.

Often these early signs are missed and people are not referred for assessment and diagnosis until there is a more dramatic change. In people with Down's syndrome this can often be when the person develops late onset seizures. Not everyone with Down's syndrome and dementia will develop these seizures, though many will. It is thought that these begin about two and a half to three years after the onset of the condition. It is often at this point that medical intervention highlights the other changes that have occurred. It is, of course, an area of concern that this is the point of referral as it means that much time has been lost in applying for increased resources and also that staff have not had the information that would enable them to respond appropriately to someone with dementia. The consequences of this often result in the person with dementia being treated as 'stubborn', 'challenging' and 'difficult' because staff misinterpret the meaning and motivation for their behaviour. It can also result in staff behaviour and responses that exacerbate the impact of the condition. (This is dealt with in Chapter 4 on working with different realities and Chapter 7 on challenging behaviour.)

The progression and characteristics of the condition will vary from person to person. Amongst people with a learning disability from causes other than Down's syndrome, the length of time that the person has the condition may be the same as the duration within the general population. For Alzheimer's disease, for example, this would be between eight and fifteen years. For people with Down's syndrome there will be a more rapid progression than in the general population; usually the progression will be from four to seven and a half years (Prasher 2005).

At the moment the time between diagnosis and death is about three to five years. This is not necessarily the length of time the person has the condition but is often the consequence of a delay in obtaining a diagnosis. This issue is dealt with fully in Chapter 3.

Summary

Dementia is an umbrella term that covers many different conditions. The most common dementias such as Alzheimer's type dementia, vascular dementia and Lewy body dementia are the conditions most likely to be encountered by those working with people with a learning disability.

People with a learning disability from causes other than Down's syndrome appear to be at higher risk of developing dementia than the general population. Research findings disagree on the extent of the risk. There is also a need for further research to differentiate between the different conditions and syndromes responsible for the learning disability. It may be that some groups are at higher risk than others or even that some conditions provide immunity.

People with Down's syndrome are at significantly higher risk of the early onset of Alzheimer's type dementia. This is thought to be linked to the fact that people with Down's syndrome have three rather than two chromosome 21. Chromosome 21 is the chromosome that is responsible for the production of beta-amyloid protein that is found in the plaques and tangles characteristic of Alzheimer's type dementia.

Amongst people with a learning disability from causes other than Down's syndrome the length of time that the person has the condition may be the same as the duration within the general population. For Alzheimer's disease, for example, this would be between eight and fifteen years. For people with Down's syndrome there will be a more rapid progression than in the general population; usually the progression will be from four to seven and a half years.

3

Getting a Diagnosis

Case study 2

Helen has a learning disability. She had lived with her parents before moving into supported housing at the age of 42. Helen had many skills before moving and had subsequently developed many more. She had become more sociable and she developed a relationship with Alan, who attended the same day service. They would both travel to events together and shared many interests. Helen was able to make simple meals for them both. Alan was keen for them to move in together but Helen was not sure about this.

There was some concern that Alan might be pressurising her. Alan began to comment on Helen's forgetfulness and that she had some problems with remembering where things were. The staff who supported her also began to notice problems in her dressing, particularly the order and type of clothes she put on. She became anxious and sometimes aggressive when there was a lot going on in the house and at the day centre. These changes were attributed to the onset of the menopause, the stresses around her relationship and her need to have more personal space. After six months of these changes being commented on, it was decided that perhaps she had the early signs of dementia; a decision was made to refer her for an assessment and to seek a diagnosis.

After some months' wait Helen was seen by a psychologist, who carried out a baseline assessment. A date six months later was set for a return assessment when any possible deterioration from the baseline would be noted and a possible diagnosis of dementia given.

The case study of Helen highlights many of the issues that are involved in obtaining an assessment and diagnosis. The main issues are:

- differential diagnosis
- delay in referral for diagnosis
- baseline information and diagnosis.

Differential diagnosis

It is possible for someone to exhibit all the early signs that are associated with dementia but not to have the condition. There are other conditions that can present like dementia. It is critical, therefore, that there is not an immediate assumption that the changed behaviours are an indication of dementia. It is essential that a process be undertaken to differentiate possible causes of the changes. This process of differential diagnosis should identify and possibly eliminate other, often treatable, conditions.

Wilkinson *et al.* (2004) found that when staff had previous experience of someone with dementia there was a tendency for them to view the changed behaviours as certain evidence of the onset of dementia. It is essential that staff are encouraged and guided to think of dementia only once other potential explanations have been eliminated.

Many conditions can trigger an acute confusional state in older people with a learning disability. People with Down's syndrome may experience this from their forties onwards. An acute confusional state will cause the person to exhibit many of the changes that are similar to those caused by dementia.

There are many common causes of acute confusional states. The following paragraphs provide information about conditions to which people with a learning disability, and especially older people with a learning disability, are particularly vulnerable. These conditions might be the cause of acute confusional states.

Endocrine or metabolic disturbance

People with Down's syndrome are particularly susceptible to hypo/ hyperthyroidism. The prevalence increases with age (Mani 1988; Prasher 1999). High levels of obesity and general overweight amongst people with a learning disability may contribute to higher levels of diabetes. Robertson *et al.* (2000) reported high levels of diabetes mellitus amongst people with Prader-Willi syndrome.

Toxicity

Toxicity can result from taking the wrong drugs, a combination of a number of drugs (polypharmacy) or just as a result of the ageing process, which means that people react to drugs that previously were tolerated.

Heart disease

Non-atherosclerotic heart disorders are more common amongst older people with a learning disability than amongst age-matched, non-disabled peers (Kapell *et al.* 1998).

Bone fractures

Fractured hips are a common cause of an acute confusional state.

Constipation

Constipation affects about 50 per cent of ambulatory and 85 per cent of non-ambulatory older people with a learning disability (Evenhuis 1997). Anti-epileptic medication may be implicated in some of the constipation experienced.

Poor diet

A poor diet may cause a deficiency in essential minerals and vitamins, particularly iron, which will lead to anaemia. Poor diet may be the consequence of poor dental health. People with a learning disability are more susceptible to dental decay and gum disease (Cumella *et al.* 2000). The consequence of poor or inconsistent dental care earlier in life has a major impact in older age (Naidu *et al.* 2001) and can lead to poor nutrition.

Dehydration

Adults should drink at least one and a half litres of fluid a day. People with a learning disability may be using a number of services and have different support staff throughout the day. There may be no record of their fluid intake.

Lack of sleep

People with Down's syndrome often have sleep apnoea, a breathing irregularity, which means that they do not get enough sleep.

Visual and hearing impairment

Older people with a learning disability have a higher rate of sensory impairment than age-matched peers in the general population (Evenhuis 1995; Kapell *et al.* 1998; Van Schrojenstein *et al.* 2000). People with Down's syndrome are particularly susceptible to cataracts (Haargaard and Fledelius 2006). Visual impairment in people with a learning disability is often the result of poor ophthalmic care throughout their lives. For a variety of reasons most will not have had eye tests. People with a learning disability may also have increased problems with hearing loss. People with a learning disability are twice as likely to have impacted ear wax as the general ageing population (Fransman 2005). This is partly caused by the reduction in the ability to chew amongst many people with a learning disability who do not have their back teeth (molars). Indeed many older people may not have any teeth. The potential for impacted ears is even greater amongst people with Down's syndrome, where a narrow ear canal predisposes them to this condition.

Environmental changes

Environmental changes can include going into hospital or moving house. Many people with a learning disability will experience multiple moves after the loss of their main carer (Oswin 1991).

Grief reactions

Grief reactions are caused by the loss of loved ones, home or health.

Pain

As people get older they are more likely to experience painful conditions such as arthritis. The prevalence of osteoporosis is higher amongst older people with a learning disability (Center, Beange and McElduff 1998; Janicki *et al.* 2002).

Multidisciplinary reviews

It is often the case that someone may have more than one of these conditions. A thorough multidisciplinary review will often reveal the complexity of the triggers. It is vital that this investigation occurs, otherwise there is a danger that one trigger is identified and because the acute confusional state remains there is the possibility of assuming that the person does indeed have an underlying dementia.

Case study 3

Paula is a woman with Down's syndrome in her early fifties. Paula's mother died after a short illness, leaving Paula alone in the house. Paula had lived with her mother all her life. After the death Paula went to stay with a sister who lived 500 miles away whilst decisions about her future were made. It was decided that Paula should return to her home town. She was moved to a supported house with four other tenants until a more permanent place could be found. Paula was eventually moved into a house with one other woman. She developed a urinary tract infection. Her eyesight was poor, a condition exacerbated by wearing dirty glasses.

Paula became very confused, aggressive, lost daily living skills and started to smell of urine. Staff supporting her, and indeed her sister, thought that she might have the early signs of dementia, which her mother had been masking, through routine and prompting support.

It is clear from closer examination of Paula's life that she had experienced loss, and change, infection and poor vision. She had an acute confusional state triggered by things that could be either cured or, with support and time, overcome.

Depression

Depression is often misdiagnosed as dementia. It can be more difficult to identify depression in some people with a learning disability because they are not able to provide classical depressive descriptions of their thoughts and feelings (Matson 1982).

Depression can look like dementia in that the person may appear to be apathetic and fail to carry out many activities of daily living. The person may appear to be losing their personal hygiene skills and may reduce their speech levels. So it is important that the depression is identified and treated appropriately.

It is not the role of direct care staff to make a diagnosis but it is important that they are aware of the role they can play in determining access to the correct interventions.

Table 3.1 on the next page has been used very successfully to raise awareness and improve practice. It is useful that this chart is reproduced in colour and preferably enlarged to A3 size. It should be displayed and made easily accessible to all staff. The table encourages staff to consider other possible explanations for changed behaviours. Only when these have been eliminated should a referral for assessment and possible diagnosis of dementia be made.

Delay in referral for diagnosis

There is something of a paradox in the area of diagnosis. On the one hand, as indicated above, there is a need to encourage staff to pull back from rushing into seeing dementia too readily. On the other hand, there is a need to get a diagnosis as soon as possible. Unfortunately there are still many delays in getting a diagnosis. Indeed diagnosis is often not made until the person has had the condition for a few years. For people with Down's syndrome the length of time between diagnosis and death is generally from three to five years (Kerr 1997). This short time span is not necessarily a true reflection of the speed of progression of the condition. It is apparent that many people with a learning disability will have had dementia for some time before a diagnosis is made. There are a number of reasons for this delay:

- problems with detection
- inexperience and lack of knowledge amongst some professionals
- unrecognised and unrecorded increase in prompting amongst carers
- denial
- carers and staff fears about the consequences of diagnosis.

Table 3.1 Procedure for investigating possible dementia in people with learning disabilities

If you notice the following changes:

- Decline in abilities and loss of skills
- Deterioration in personality or behaviour
- Poor memory and confusion

then you should consider all the following

	Symptoms	Actions
Stress	Concentration problems Irritability Decline in abilities	Identify stressor Recent life events e.g. death, a move, illness Offer support and reassurance
Thyroid	Lethargy Weight gain Cold intolerance Changes in skin and hair	See GP Annual blood tests Under or over active thyroid Medication
Depression	Disturbed sleep Loss of appetite Low mood Withdrawal from usual activities Tearful	See GP Medication and/or counselling
Sensory Impairment	Ignores instructions Mobility problems Loss of confidence Shouting or raised voice	Complete full health surveillance Check: eyes, ears, feet Access appropriate services
Physical Causes	Withdrawal Aggression Self-injury Pacing Screaming Crying	See GP Medical history and physical investigations Medication changes Diabetes Pain Urinary tract infection Nutritional deficiencies/dehydration
Dementia	Loss of recent memory Loss of skills Changes in mood Orientation difficulties Sleep disturbances Language difficulties	Refer to Community Learning Disabilities Team (CLDT) Follow on referral to appropriate clinicians e.g. GP, psychology, neurology, occupational therapy, speech and language therapy, physiotherapy

Source: Earnshaw and Donnelly (2001)

Problems with detection

A look at the list of early signs of the onset of dementia will reveal that many of the manifestations are often already present amongst people with a learning disability. People may already have memory problems, poor concentration, difficulty with daily living skills, communication problems and poor orientation. This can sometimes mean that it is difficult to detect the deterioration. Where the changes are noticed they are sometimes simply attributed to the learning disability, or to the person 'being stubborn' or just 'getting older'. It is critical that the changes are recorded, as it is not the existence of these characteristics but the changes in them that are significant for diagnosis.

Inexperience and lack of knowledge amongst some professionals

The increased longevity experienced by people with a learning disability means that professionals now have to deal with issues of older age. This puts many at a disadvantage as their training may well have concentrated on younger age issues. The opportunities, until recently, to be involved with older people with a learning disability have been limited. This is exacerbated for some professionals who do not specialise in the field of learning disability and so their caseloads involve many different client and patient groups. This is particularly the case for many general practitioners (GPs) who, despite the fact that 'general practitioners are the health professionals most commonly consulted by people with intellectual disability' (Lennox and Eastgate 2004, p.601), will have only a limited experience of people with a learning disability as they constitute a small proportion of any GP's list (National Health Service (NHS) Scotland 2004). A study carried out in Glasgow found that on average each GP would have only five people with a learning disability registered with them (Glasgow University Affiliated Department 2002).

Most GPs will have limited experience of people with dementia even within the general population. 'A GP with 1,500 to 2000 patients can expect to include 12–20 people with dementia, depending on the age profile of the list' (Alzheimer's Disease Society 1995, p. 2). The amount of experience that any one GP will have of people with a learning disability who also have dementia therefore is going to be fairly limited. This inevitably will have an impact on the recognition of possible dementia and the need for referral for assessment (Wilkinson *et al.* 2004).

Unrecognised and unrecorded increase in prompting amongst carers

Case study 4

Jonathan had always needed a verbal prompt to remind him to do his teeth each morning. Over the past weeks the staff member supporting him had noticed that he responded better to a visual prompt. She had, as well as telling him to do his teeth, used the visual prompt of showing him his toothbrush. Jonathan has had to be prompted to remind him to take his coat off when he arrives at the day service; previously he had taken it off straight away and put it on his peg. He has also been found wandering around the centre. On enquiry staff found he wanted the toilet. A staff member walked along with him prompting him to help him find the way. At night when it is his turn to do the tea, Jonathan, who used to find everything in the cupboards easily, now hesitates when looking for certain china. A staff member prompts him in the right direction.

Jonathan's declining skills are being continuously and immediately compensated for. But no one is recording the various prompts, and the cumulative effect and significance is lost.

People supporting those with a learning disability will be involved in providing prompts to help them accomplish the tasks of daily living. Getting the right level of prompting is, of course, critical to facilitate independence and enhance self-esteem. The onset of dementia leads inevitably to a decline in skills. Staff and carers, however, will often absorb and compensate for these changes by increasing their prompting. This is the correct response but unfortunately often the increases are not noticed, or if they are they are not seen as significant. As Chris Oliver (1998, p. 124) points out, people with a learning disability are 'likely to be in services in which a care culture is prominent … deficits acquired over time may simply be absorbed … in the same way that deficits of adaptive behaviour … are managed'. Caring, supporting and prompting are what good carers and staff do. The danger is that they are not sufficiently aware of what is happening and consequently miss the significance of what they are doing.

Many people with a learning disability will, during the course of one day, require support from a number of people. One staff member may not think that his or her extra prompt is significant, but if a formal record is kept by everyone involved the extent of the increased support will be evidenced and help to build a picture of what is happening.

The record of prompting chart provides an example of the type of record that could be kept (Table 3.2).

Table 3.2 Record of prompting chart

Person's name:

Task: being supported to shave

Score key: 0=independently; 1=verbal prompt; 2=physical promt; 3=do task for person; 4=person did not want to do task

Prompt	Score/Date/ Staff initials	Score/Date/ Staff initials	Score/Date/ Staff initials
Prompt to put plug in	1 15/02/04 DK		
Prompt to run hot/cold water	2		
Check temperature of water	3		
Prompt to open foam	1		
Prompt to apply foam	2		
Prompt to wet razor	1		
Prompt to shave	2		
Left side of face	2		
Right side of face	2		
Under chin	2		
Below mouth	3		
Below nose	3		
Prompt to look in mirror	3		
Repeat above if needed	1		
Prompt to wash off foam	0		
Prompt to dry face	0		

Source: Adapted from Cairns and Kerr (1994)

Denial

Many staff will have chosen to work within the learning disability service because they want to be part of enabling people to reach their potential. They will find reward in being part of a team that enables people to grow, develop skills and gain an increased sense of self-worth. Close attachments are often formed; sometimes staff will have known the person they support for many years. It can be hard, therefore, for them to accept that the gains that they have been part of and witnessed are being lost.

Similarly parents and siblings will often find it difficult to acknowledge that their family member is declining in skills. This can be particularly distressing for parents who have previously worried that they will experience declining skills and death before their adult child and have now to review the possibility that the order may be reversed.

Carer and staff fears about the consequences of diagnosis

I have often been told by carers that they did not want to alert the authorities to the possibility that their son or daughter might have dementia because they felt that all the hard-won gains that had been achieved would be removed. There is a fear that the person with dementia will lose their day service place, their place in a supported house or tenancy and be placed in a residential or nursing home for older people. This was expressed by the mother of one man who stated: 'I have fought hard all his life to get the support he now has. I am not going to rock the boat by suggesting that he might have dementia'.

This worry is mirrored by support staff (Wilkinson, Kerr and Cunningham 2005). Staff have often had the experience of someone with dementia being placed in an old people's residential or nursing home and usually this has not been perceived as a good experience. It is seen as something to be avoided. One way to avoid this is to delay the seeking of a diagnosis.

These perceptions, whether correct or not, can sometimes hinder referral for assessment and diagnosis.

Baseline information and diagnosis

Making a referral does not necessarily lead to an easy and speedy diagnosis. Staff are often not clear who to refer to and when. The lack of a clear 'pathway' impedes the process. Service providers need to develop diagnostic pathways that are made clear and accessible to all staff. The route or pathway will depend on where the expertise lies, numbers being referred, people's own interests and, of course, geography and resources. The peculiarities of pathways mean that it is essential to be clear who is responsible for what and when and how they need to be approached. Staff will often ask fundamental questions about whom they should approach about their worries. If staff do not know where to start, then referral will be delayed.

Further delay in diagnosis can occur if there is a lack of baseline information. For people without a learning disability there is a standard test that is given if there is a suspicion of dementia. This test, the Mini Mental State Examination (MMSE), assumes a level of competence against which loss of ability can be measured. This test is, inevitably, unsuitable for people with a learning disability who would never have achieved the 'normal' score or indeed in most cases would not achieve the score that indicates the possible existence of dementia. For some people there will be a floor effect, where their own 'normal' score would have been at the bottom of the MMSE scale. For these reasons the MMSE is not a suitable tool for diagnosing dementia in people with a learning disability. This then presents a potential difficulty. Before any diagnosis can be made it is essential to determine the individual's baseline abilities. It is only by measuring deterioration against the individual's normal baseline score that dementia can be indicated.

Psychologists and others involved in assessment and diagnosis often use a series of different tools in combination to determine baseline information and to measure the changes. There is no single preferred or generally used set of tools and people often struggle to determine which tools to use as well as how and when in the process. The Cambridge Examination for Mental Disorders of Older People with Down's Syndrome and Others with Intellectual Disabilities (CAMDEX-DS) may simplify this process. This pack comprises a series of tools that can be used by various professionals to provide essential information to be used in the diagnostic process and the development of individual care plans (Ball *et al.* 2006).

The problems of determining a baseline assessment mean that the process of diagnosis will necessitate the carrying out of a series of tests to establish the person's range of abilities. There will then be a delay and a follow-up assessment will be carried out six months or more later. This delay can be considerably shortened by the development of baseline information prior to the onset of dementia.

For people with Down's syndrome it is advisable to develop formal baseline assessments from the age of 30 if possible, but certainly from the age of 35. The assessments should then be carried out at decreasing intervals as the person ages (Oliver 1998). For people with a learning disability with causes other than Down's syndrome, because generally there is a later age of onset of the condition it is not necessary to carry out the baseline assessment until later. It is important that the baseline information is carried out within a general health-screening programme. It should not be carried out as an isolated intervention, which may then require an explanation as to why the person has been singled out for this particular assessment.

Fife multidisciplinary health-screening clinic for clients with Down's syndrome

This is an example of an award-winning programme that integrated the process into general health screening.

The West Fife CLDT developed the health-screening clinic for people with Down's syndrome in November 2004. The clinic aims to provide a comprehensive screening programme for all individuals with Down's syndrome in one locality, via involvement from various members of the CLDT. A 'one-stop shop' format is adopted, where the client attends for one appointment and is seen by all members of the team for a varied range of assessments. During the clinic the departments of nursing, psychology, speech and language therapy, physiotherapy, podiatry and dietetics carry out assessments. The full screening normally takes around two hours to complete, but the atmosphere is relaxed, with refreshments available throughout. The appropriate professionals follow up any issues that are detected in the clinic, and the GP is notified of the clinic findings. Where no issues are identified, the information gathered acts as a baseline measurement against which future findings can be compared. The health-screening clinics run on a monthly basis with clients over the age of 35 invited to be reviewed annually, and those under 35 invited every two years.

This CLDT programme was set up specifically for people with Down's syndrome. It could be adapted to encompass people with a learning disability with other causes. The screening and baseline assessments for dementia would not then need to be carried out until a much later age because of the later onset in comparison to people with Down's syndrome.

The importance of keeping information

Systematically gathered and recorded information about an individual's skills, abilities and behaviours can provide important background and evidence for the person doing the assessment and diagnosis. Services should identify and consistently use a tool to record this information. The tool chosen should require minimum training for carers and ensure the recording of consistent, coherent and meaningful information on dementia-specific behaviours. The information is usually readily available but not necessarily recorded. Staff will know a great deal about the person they support. They need to make sure that this is not just kept in their heads. The psychology service can be approached for further information on the use of suitable tools and training.

The development of life story work, as described in Chapter 6 on therapeutic interventions, can play an important role in the process of diagnosis. Knowing about someone's past life can provide details and information that could explain the changes in behaviour that may be indicative of dementia. If people return to behaviours that they have abandoned, this may indicate that they have lost more recent memory and feel more 'at home' doing things from their past.

Magnetic resonance imaging (MRI) scanning

Sometimes the person doing the assessment will want to defer diagnosis until a brain scan has been carried out. This is particularly problematic for most people with a learning disability. The scan involves the person being restricted to a confined space, which can cause immense stress and anxiety. This will often necessitate the use of sedation.

A study carried out to investigate whether the use of MRI scanning could detect Alzheimer's disease in adults with Down's syndrome (Prasher *et al.* 2003) had to be terminated because of the high risk of medical complications related to sedation. Out of the 38 subjects, three developed respiratory complications after the application of intravenous sedation.

Within the study, which had 19 people with Down's syndrome and Alzheimer's disease and 19 with Down's syndrome but without Alzheimer's disease, only 8 people were compliant with testing without sedation, 16 were compliant with sedation, 6 had poor compliance with sedation and 8 people were completely non-compliant even with sedation. The conclusion of the research was that 'magnetic resonance imaging (MRI) has an important but limited role to play in the management of Alzheimer's disease in the population with Down's syndrome. If intravenous sedation is used, medical support is essential to prevent a serious mishap' (Prasher *et al.* 2003, p. 90). So it is fair to say that extreme caution should be exercised in the pursuit of MRI scanning as a diagnostic tool for dementia in the learning disabled population.

Summary

There are many conditions that can trigger changes that can easily be confused with dementia. It is critical that a differential diagnosis is carried out to determine if the changes are the result of the onset of an acute confusional state, delirium or depression. Once these have been eliminated as possible explanations then it is essential that a referral for an assessment for possible dementia be obtained as soon as possible. There are, however, a number of reasons why there is often a considerable delay in the making of the necessary referral.

Because the person has a learning disability, there can be a problem with detection. The person may already have deficits in the areas that would indicate the presence of dementia. Amongst some professionals, GPs for example, there may be a lack of experience of people with a learning disability and particularly of people with a learning disability and dementia. There are also unrecognised and so unrecorded increases in prompting by those supporting the person. The cumulative effect of the increase in prompting across the various services and personnel is often not recognised early on in the development of the condition. There is also an element of denial by those who have been involved with the support and care of someone who they have seen develop and flourish. The possibility that they may be developing a condition that will strip them of their gains, and ultimately of their life, can lead staff and carers to search for other explanations. There can also exist a fear amongst staff and families that an acknowledgement of the onset of the condition might lead to withdrawal of services and the move of the person to another setting.

Once a referral has been made, there can be a considerable delay in obtaining a diagnosis. One important reason for this is the lack of baseline information. This lack will necessitate the person having a formal assessment of abilities and then a delay of up to a year to see if their condition deteriorates from this position. The implementation of baseline assessments prior to the onset of the condition is essential. For people with Down's syndrome, these should commence in their early thirties.

4

Working with Different Realities

To understand the difficulties that people with dementia experience in relation to their memory and understanding of where they are, what they are doing and who they and others are, it is necessary to understand some of the ways in which memory is stored and subsequently damaged by the dementia.

We have two kinds of memory, short-term and long-term memory. New information is stored in our short-term memory for about 20–30 seconds before being transported into our long-term memory. This is not an automatic process. Whether we retain information by moving it back into our long-term memory depends on the way the information is given, received and experienced. It also requires us to work at it. We need to pay attention and concentrate. Another influencing factor is the emotional content of the information or event. The more emotionally significant the more likely it is to become embedded in our memory. Repetition of information, events and skills will aid retention and seeing information or being able to visualise it significantly aids the storing of information. The use of association is also important. We can remember something if we can 'hang' the information on to something else that we can associate it with, and of course the more meaningful the information the more chance there is that it will be retained in our memory.

When someone develops dementia, even if the above conditions apply, the ability to retain the memory and move it back into the long-term memory becomes increasingly disturbed and eventually lost. From the time of the onset of the dementia, therefore, the amount of new information stored will be diminished.

As the dementia progresses, even information and events that are stored in the long-term memory will begin to disappear. Huub Buijssen (2005) describes and illustrates this process through the idea of diaries. He describes our memory as stored in diaries, one for each year of our life. People without dementia will have all their diaries stored chronologically and intact on the shelf.

If we imagine a shelf of diaries, one diary for each year of our life, then with the onset of dementia memories begin to get lost and a domino effect takes place with the diaries slowly falling down. Only those left standing will have meaning and memory for the person (see Figure 4.1). Buijssen describes this as roll-back memory.

The memory of a 77-year-old without dementia – the shelf on which the diaries containing the memories of his entire life are stacked is still intact.

Years

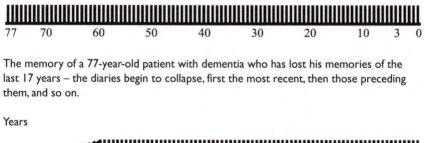

The memory of a 77-year-old patient with dementia who has lost his memories of the last 17 years – the diaries begin to collapse, first the most recent, then those preceding them, and so on.

Years

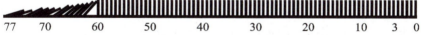

The memory of someone in the advanced stage of dementia – only the memories of his early childhood remain.

Years

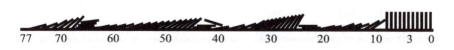
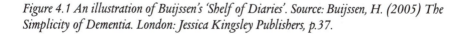

Figure 4.1 An illustration of Buijssen's 'Shelf of Diaries'. Source: Buijssen, H. (2005) The Simplicity of Dementia. London: Jessica Kingsley Publishers, p.37.

When the part of the brain that hold short-term and recent memory is damaged then the person will make sense of information and stimuli in that part of the brain that is functioning. As illustrated by Buijssen's diaries this will be the brain that holds earlier memories. New information will be made sense of within the 'diaries' that remain. The person's sense of reality will not be in the here and now, in our reality, but the there and then, their past.

I often illustrate this point in relation to my own possible reactions to developing dementia and being moved to live in a home for older people in later life. Part of my job is to visit homes for older people and to train staff. This means that I am often in homes for older people where the staff are sitting around listening attentively, with occasional discussion and conversation.

If I develop dementia in later life and find myself in a home for older people I will make sense of my environment in relation to my past rather than the then present. To be in a home where people are sitting around often not speaking will present a well-known and well-understood scenario. I will believe that I am there to train the staff. The long-term memory part of my brain will interpret all the immediate information and stimuli making sense of them in my long-term memory and this will confirm that I am the teacher and certainly not a resident. What of course is almost unbearable is the realisation that as a teacher I would reasonably expect to go home at the end of the afternoon. To be told that 'this is your home now' would be both incredible and terrifying.

People with dementia are making sense of the world around them using the brain that is functioning, which increasingly involves the use of long-term rather than the short-term memory. This means that often they perceive and understand the world from a different time and place and therefore will have a different reality. This difference can be and often is a source of immense anxiety and fear for people with dementia. The following exercise illustrates this point well.

Imagine you set off from your house to your local pub to meet your friends. You always go as soon as your favourite soap on the television is over; in fact the tune at the end is the signal for you to put your coat on. On the way there, two people come up to you and take you by the arm and refuse to let you go on any further. They insist on you going with them. Imagine what you might feel, what might you think was going on? What might you do and say? It is not hard to imagine the panic and fear that this might engender.

Because the brain is damaged and cognitive skills diminished, the 'trigger' of the music ending the television soap results in the person re-enacting past behaviours and realities. People from the present become unrecognisable. They did not exist in the past. The dementia means that people begin to lose the ability to recognise the familiar. They will see the world as a foreign place peopled by strangers (Meisen 1993). This can happen even when they remain at home surrounded by people they have known for many years and who are caring and supportive of them. It is not just a consequence of being moved into different settings such as hospitals or residential or nursing homes.

Of course the desire to be in the past may also be psychologically functional. If the present is full of fear, anxiety and an assault on the sense of self it may be safer to be in the past. It is important to see the 'not being in the here and now' as a function not simply of the changes in the brain but of a complex dynamic between the physical, social and psychological changes and needs of the person with dementia.

This characteristic of dementia can present those supporting people with difficulties, as the following case study illustrates.

Case study 5

Mary is a woman aged 56 with Down's syndrome and a diagnosis of dementia. Mary has recently started to announce every morning that she cannot stay (in her supported house where she has been for 12 years), as she has to get home to help her mummy walk the dogs. Mary's mother died not long after she moved into her supported accommodation.

There are a number of responses to Mary's statement. First, it is crucial that the meaning and motivation behind her statements are considered. If we are going to respond appropriately to people with dementia, we must try to understand the motivation and meaning that informs their behaviour.

Is Mary saying that she wants to go home because she feels lost, frightened and insecure and wants to be where she knows things will be secure and safe? The expression 'Home is where the heart is' is relevant here. Maybe she does not any longer feel her heart is in her present accommodation. Her desire to be with her mother may well be triggered by a sense of anxiety and loss. The need to be mothered is strong when we feel alone and lost and insecure.

It may well be that Mary's mention of 'home' and 'mother', two very emotive words and anchors in most people's lives, is an expression of her feelings and not an actual statement about what needs to happen. It could also be a clear and unequivocal statement about the facts as she now sees them. If she now believes that she is 25 again, then of course she will believe that she needs to hurry to get the dogs walked as she did for many years throughout her teens.

Clearly the worker needs to respond here with intelligent understanding and great sensitivity to reduce Mary's anxiety and avoid increasing her stress.

There are three options in cases like Mary's:

- using reality orientation
- using a validation techniques
- telling a lie.

Using reality orientation

Reality orientation means finding ways to orientate people to reality. People who work with and support people with a learning disability will be familiar with these techniques, even if this is not the term used. People will use a variety of visual and conversational cues to help people orientate themselves in time and place.

An example would be the way in which staff might use a picture board with days of the week on it to remind someone when they go to their day service. If someone repeatedly insists that their brother is going to visit them soon, even though their brother has moved to Australia, the worker may gently remind the person of their brother's move. Pictures and letters sent from Australia would help to reinforce the reality. This is good and constructive use of reality orientation.

Reality orientation has been transferred to work with people with dementia. Its use, however, is not straightforward. The purpose has to be to enable people to retain control, as far as possible, to reduce stress and facilitate their hold on reality, if this is what is in their best interest.

Unfortunately reality orientation is often used where it has the opposite impact of these desired outcomes.

> To remind Mary that her mother is dead, that she is now 65 and there are no dogs to be walked would certainly tell her about reality but to what purpose? If Mary says that her mother is waiting for her, then for Mary her mother exists. To remind her of the truth would be to plummet her into grief. Mary would be pulled into a world that reminds her of her loss. She has dementia and so short-term memory loss. She will forget the 'truth' she has been told but will be left with the feeling of loss and anxiety that may well remain with her throughout the day. Then next day she will again say she needs to walk the dogs. What has been gained? Nothing but distress for Mary.

It is concerning that such practice still occurs and, indeed, is sometimes encouraged by practitioners who insist that we must not 'collude with false reality'. This notion comes from the field of psychiatric work with people with particular psychiatric illnesses and has no place in work with people with dementia. To tell someone with dementia the truth when it is going to cause immense stress and grief is cruel and unacceptable.

This is not to refute the correct use of reality orientation with people with dementia. It certainly has a place, particularly in the early stages when people are 'nearly orientated' (Chapman, Jacques and Marshall 1994). People will often benefit from gentle reminders that help them orientate. The type of reminders and cues need to be thought through on an individual basis. For people with a learning disability, the use of written material may be already considerably limited so the use of pictures and photos is often a better option. Using orientating cues in the conversation can be equally effective. Saying 'today is Wednesday … on Wednesday we go to …' will orientate to the day especially if the day is repeated. Reality orientation is most useful when it is embedded in significant relationships and is a thread running through people's lives.

The use of group activities to enable reality orientation can provide stimulation and encourage the person to engage with the world around them but this must be a meaningful and stress-free activity. There must be constant monitoring to guard against over-stimulation. It must also be recognised that the person might not want to be orientated to a reality where there is a world that feels unsafe, lonely and frightening.

Using validation techniques

This is a way of working that gives validity to the person with dementia's perception of reality. It respects their need to feel in control and unthreatened. Naomi Feil (1992) has written extensively on the use of validation as a therapy to 'help the disorientated old'. Her work does not solely focus on people with dementia and has aspects that are not relevant to people with a learning disability and dementia. The philosophy that underpins her work and some of the techniques she advocates are relevant, however, and indeed crucial to working with people with dementia whose reality is changing. It can certainly be used therapeutically with people with dementia. It is in essence a way of relating and communicating that requires the person without dementia to step into the reality of the person with dementia, to walk in their shoes. The technique requires us to listen to what the person with dementia is saying and to pick up on their concerns, needs, feelings and reality as they express them. Naomi Feil writes that 'validation uses empathy to tune into the inner reality of the disorientated [person]. Empathy ... builds trust. Trust brings safety. Safety brings strength. Strength renews feelings of worth. Worth reduces stress. ... And restores dignity' (Feil 1992, pp. 10–11).

> To return to Mary: a way of validating her reality would be to say, 'Wait whilst I get my coat and I will walk down the street with you'. This is not saying that you are taking her to her mother, it is simply engaging with her need to leave. It is a way of empathising with her feelings of not 'being at home' or of 'wanting her mummy'. Often in such instances the walk outside will prove distracting. It is hoped that the attention she receives will counteract her feelings of being alone and lost. Mary will forget what triggered her need to 'go home' and a suggestion that 'perhaps the kettle is boiling by now' may be sufficient to get her to return.
>
> Another option would be to engage with Mary in talking about the dogs: 'Where did you go for walks?' 'How old were the dogs?' 'What were their names?' etc. Talking about the dogs may well allow her to feel that she is being taken seriously. The need for the dogs to be acknowledged will be met. Mary has a short-term memory deficit. If she can have her agitation reduced she will forget the cause of it and can then be distracted and diverted onto other things.

The person with dementia may perceive themselves as being much younger. They may well be at the stage when they could reasonably expect their mother to be around and certainly that their home is still there. It is also worth acknowledging the fact that people with dementia use the terms 'mother' and 'home' probably more than any other emotive words. We convey our reality through words. The worker must attend to the implications the use of these words has for understanding the reality of the person with dementia.

In Chapter 5 on communication the significance of the use of the idea of 'home' and 'mother' is explored in the context of what the person might be trying to communicate. In terms of different realities it is important to consider the meaning behind these words.

I am often asked why people with a learning disability and dementia who have been in long-stay hospital for much of their life and have seen little of their mother or home, still say that they must go home to their mummy. Perhaps an answer is that the child who is separated from the mother is the child who is always waiting for their mother to come and get them, to make it all better and take them home. As the dementia progresses the person may return to that period in their life when they waited and hoped for such an event.

Telling a lie

To lie does of course present an ethical dilemma. We should not be lying to people. This option should be considered only if it is the only way to avoid stressing the person. It is possible that a statement such as 'The dogs have already been for their walk today' might deal with the problem. It might, on the other hand, make Mary angry that someone had done her job.

The problem with telling an untruth, apart from the obvious ethical dilemma, is that people with dementia will have times of increased lucidity. They may remember that you lied and this would be damaging to your relationship.

The debate here is no different from the one that would pertain to the telling of 'white lies' in our daily lives when we may chose to tell an untruth if it would save someone from unnecessary hurt and anxiety. The decision is not an easy one. As with other interventions this should not be a decision left to individual staff members but should be discussed, reviewed and embedded in good, coherent and consistent practice.

It is important to know that there are no absolute answers. What might be right in one situation with one person may be wrong in another situation with a different person. In trying to decide on a response the person and the context must be considered.

Removal of stimuli

It would also be useful to consider what might be triggering the need to walk the dogs. If it is to do with the light fading, a television programme or something else, this should be identified and either eliminated from the environment or Mary distracted beforehand. These ideas are expanded upon in Chapter 7 on challenging behaviour and Chapter 11 on the environment.

Summary

The damage caused to the brain by the onset of dementia means that people will begin to lose their short-term memory and will increasingly experience the world with the part of the brain that contains their long-term memories. They will experience themselves as younger and will forget events and people in the more recent past. Increasingly they will return to their childhood memories. The consequence is that their reality becomes different from ours. It is important to remember that their reality is as real to them as ours is to us. To contradict their perception will often cause undue stress and even grief. This must be avoided at all cost. There are three options for carers in dealing with this phenomenon. The use of reality orientation can be employed to remind the person of the present: this is acceptable only if it does not distress the person. Validation can be used: this involves stepping into the person's shoes and acknowledging their reality, walking beside them and, when appropriate, distracting and diverting them to something else. Lastly there is the possibility of telling an untruth: this raises a number of moral and practical dilemmas and should be considered only if it is the only way to avoid stressing the person.

5

Maintaining Good Communication

The onset of dementia will usually affect the part of the brain that deals with language. This means that there will now be significant and increasing deterioration in the person's level of verbal ability. The ability to both understand and use words and language becomes impaired. Additionally, because the part of the brain that we use to identify the geography of our body also becomes damaged, people who had previously used sign languages, such as Makaton, will find it harder to use them.

Sometimes it can seem that the person is cut off, perhaps talking 'rubbish' and even deliberately not communicating. It is important to remember that if those of us without dementia, whose brains are intact, find it difficult to understand the person with dementia, then how much more of a struggle must it be for the person with dementia to understand and communicate with us. It is essential that those supporting people with dementia and a learning disability know that no matter what stage of the condition they are at they still want to communicate.

People with a learning disability are likely to have had some problems with communication prior to the onset of dementia. Staff will have developed ways of helping them communicate and will themselves have developed understanding of the various communication patterns and strategies used by the person. It can be hard for staff to realise that they now need to develop new strategies and understandings.

There are a number of communication problems that might develop as the condition progresses, for example:

- *Dysarthia:* Slurred speech.

- *Aphasia:* An inability to use language or to understand the spoken word. This is especially the case with words that are not commonly used by the person or are highly abstract.

- *Agnosia:* Loss of ability to recognise objects, either by name or by sight. This will include the ability to recognise the written word or modern symbols.

- *Apraxia:* Loss of ability to form purposeful movements. This can extend to the inability to remember the patterns used to form words.

The following changes are the most commonly experienced:

- difficulties in finding words

- loss of comprehension

- poor articulation

- unusual patterns of speech

- repetition of words and phrases

- loss of ability to sign and gesture – very slight in the early stages but will increase in severity as the condition progresses

- reduction in and eventual loss of speech.

The word-finding difficulties mean that the person will often use a word that roughly describes the object – for example, a car may become 'the wheel thing' or shoes 'the foot things'. As the condition progresses, emptier words will be used so that a chair may become 'that thing' or a carer or relative 'that person'.

The need to attend to the meaning behind the words is critical. Because the person has lost the ability to find the correct words they will often use words, phrases and even music that convey their feelings and meaning obliquely. We need to resist the temptation to take words at face value. It is important to think what the feelings might be behind the communication and to try to interpret the words as an expression of a feeling and not just as a literal expression

As discussed in Chapter 4 on different realities, people with dementia express the ideas of 'mother' and 'home' often. Because it is so important to address and emphasise the issues that these ideas raise, they are discussed further in this chapter. The woman who constantly tells you her mummy is waiting for her may well be saying that she wishes her mummy was there. She may be conveying the feeling that she is lost and alone and wants 'mothering'. The person who tells you they are 'going home now' may well be saying that they feel worried and if they were at home they would be all right. The saying 'Home is where the heart is' is an important one for people to remember when supporting those with dementia. If someone says they are going home, they may be saying, 'My heart is not here, I feel alone and confused'. In these circumstances it would be wrong for staff to tell people this is your home. The only person who knows where their heart is is the person themselves. Telling someone they are already at home or indeed that their mother is dead will actually feed the feeling of distress and loneliness. We can only guess at the hidden meaning and feelings but we should pause at least and consider that the person's words may not literally convey their true intent. The following examples illustrate a useful way to help staff to engage with this process:

What is said / done?	Possible meaning	Underlying feelings
A man shouting, 'I am going home, I hate this place.'	'I need the toilet, I cannot find it but I know where it is at home.'	Worry, embarrassment, fear.
The woman who keeps asking the time.	'I want to do something else, but I need someone to help me when the time is right.'	Worry, boredom, frustration.

Telling the man that 'This is your home now' or repeatedly telling the woman the time will not address what they are really trying to communicate. Nor will it attend to their underlying feelings. The use of some of the techniques described in Chapter 4 on different realities may be a better response.

For most of us only 20 per cent of our communication is verbal while 80 per cent is non-verbal, that is touch, tone of voice, facial expression, gesture and body language. Someone with a learning disability may already have difficulty with verbal skills and so be heavily reliant on non-verbal information. This reliance is increased by the onset of dementia. With the impairment of verbal communication skills the non-verbal communication becomes even more important. People with dementia will become much more aware of the emotional content of any exchange. This can easily lead to severe communication difficulties, caused by the carer relying on verbal cues whilst the person with dementia is responding to body language and facial expression.

Case study 6

Hannah, a 49-year-old woman with a learning disability and dementia, is sitting in the hall waiting for the bus to take her to the day centre. She calls her support worker over to help her with her coat. The telephone rings and her support worker says, 'I am just going to answer the phone, Hannah, I will be back in a minute.' Hannah does not understand the words: what she knows is that her worker has turned her back, walked away and 'abandoned' her. Hannah starts to shout and pushes another tenant as he passes her. Although the worker has promised to return and help Hannah, the message Hannah has received is that she has been abandoned. The non-verbal communication has not been mitigated by the verbal reassurances.

Carers will be familiar with similar situations where their words of support or concern are not heard but the person with dementia responds to their stressed facial expression or their body language.

Staff and caregivers must be alert to the non-verbal cues and communication given by the person with dementia. Malcolm Goldsmith (1996, p.111) comments: 'it is probable that many opportunities are missed because carers are not sufficiently skilled at recognising and interpreting non verbal communication'. This tendency is probably exacerbated by the attention given within the learning disability service to behaviour that challenges. There is a danger that non-verbal behaviours in people with dementia will be seen as evidence of the extension, development or reappearance of challenging behaviour rather than the attempts of a person struggling to communicate.

It is important to remember that the person with dementia will feel increasingly out of control and confused by their environment. This will increase their stress levels and will in turn make finding the right words or phrases more difficult. It is essential, therefore, that all communication is conducted in a stress-free environment. This involves managing not only the physical environment but also our own behaviours and unintended messages.

Communication difficulties can be made worse if the person has difficulty concentrating. This will occur if there is a lot of noise in the room, if there are two conversations going on in the same room or if the person is trying to talk and walk at the same time. The lack of a hearing aid or glasses or, indeed, dirty glasses will also create a further barrier to communication. The person may not have control over these pieces of equipment. There is a possibility that diagnostic overshadowing (the tendency to attribute all the changes and losses that the person experiences to the existence of dementia) will reduce staff attention to these aids, as they attribute the communication problems solely to the impact of the condition.

The difficulties that people with dementia have in both using and understanding the spoken word require those who support them to be increasingly inventive and knowledgeable about the use of non-verbal interactions.

Touch

The use of touch as a form of non-verbal communication becomes increasingly necessary. Touch is a fundamental form of communication that we all use even when our verbal skills are intact. The struggle to find the right words, or even a complete failure to find them, leaves people potentially isolated and anxious. Touch then becomes a vital way not only of communicating that they are being attended to but also of providing comfort and security amid the stress and anxiety that goes with the increasing loss of the ability to communicate.

Many people with a learning disability and especially people with Down's syndrome will experience higher than usual levels of visual impairment and hearing loss (Kerr 1997). Inevitably these conditions impair communication. Touch becomes a way of cutting through the distance that this creates between people.

In the context of the above information and knowledge, it is of great concern that many people who support those with a learning disability and dementia are not only discouraged but also sometimes told not to touch people unless it is part of a necessary intervention. The uses of 'no hugs' policies are anathema to the needs and well-being of people with dementia. Of course there has been and still is a rightful concern about the inappropriate and abusive use of touch with people with a learning disability. Appropriate training, care planning and risk assessment should be in place to ensure that those supporting people with a learning disability and dementia are themselves taught to use touch appropriately. There must be a recognition of the role that touch plays in all our lives and especially in the lives of people whose condition leaves them alone, anxious and agitated and struggling to communicate. (See Chapter 6 on therapeutic interventions for more discussion on the use of touch as a therapeutic intervention.)

Music

It is an often-observed phenomenon that people with dementia who have increasing difficulty finding the right words to express themselves will sing an entire song (Rainbow 2003). This is something that caregivers should build on and use as a means of communication (the use of music as a specific therapeutic intervention is discussed in Chapter 6 on therapeutic interventions). People will often sing a song that reflects their mood or even expresses something they want to convey. They may play an instrument loudly or bang drums hard or play softly as an expression of their mood. Clair (1996, p. 73) suggests that 'people with dementia may even use music as an iconic representation of the feelings they can no longer express in words'. Staff should listen to the song or the instrumental expression and determine, if possible, if there is a message being conveyed.

Equally staff should sing to the person with dementia. If you join in when they are singing you are communicating with them. You are making it clear that you are 'in tune with them', that you can hear them and that you are giving them time. This communicates much that the use of the spoken word will fail to do.

Things that will aid good verbal communication

Touch and music are examples of ways in which non-verbal communication can be enhanced. However, there will be times when speech is possible, appropriate and necessary no matter how distorted the person's words and sentences are.

When communicating verbally there are a number of practical things that can be used to reduce problems and enhance communication with the person with dementia. The following list provides some useful suggestions on what to avoid doing:

- Don't use abstract or metaphorical language – for example, 'It's raining cats and dogs'.
- Don't use long complicated sentences with unnecessary detail.
- Don't rush the person.
- Don't correct the person's communication attempts.
- Don't expect the person to understand the first time round.
- Don't introduce new words, signs or symbols.
- Don't address the person when you are busy doing something else or when the environment is busy.

Here are some suggestions for facilitating good verbal communication:

- Find a quiet calming place to talk.
- Do get the person's attention before communicating with them e.g. use their name, touch their arm (if tolerated), reduce distractions and ensure good lighting.
- Approach the person from the front. Make sure that you establish eye contact before you touch them.
- Smile when you are sure you have been seen.
- Identify yourself and use their name.
- Try to talk to the person on your own.
- Work out when the person is most able to concentrate and understand you, and if possible communicate important things then (remember that the effects of dementia vary during the day).
- Speak a little more slowly and as clearly as possible.
- Use words, signs and concrete objects that are familiar to the person.
- There must be consistency across the staff group in the use of terminology and order of words.

- Give lots of reminders when you are giving information. For example, 'Your brother Bill is coming today', 'Bill will take you out'.

- Give the person time to respond.

- Prompt and gently remind them of the topic if they wander off. But do not insist.

- Keep questions simple and ask only one at a time.

- Do make sure that if the person is wearing a hearing aid that it is turned on. Also make sure that their glasses are clean.

- Use visual cues such as photos.

- Allow and encourage the person to talk about the past. This is very often easier for someone with dementia.

- Be encouraging.

- Use touch appropriately.

- Use music: singing is an excellent form of communication.

Summary

Communication will already be an area of difficulty for many people with a learning disability. The onset of dementia exacerbates this. The person will experience a decline in whatever communication skills they had and will become increasingly dependent on other forms of communication. Non-verbal forms of communication will need to be increased as will the use of touch and music. Communication should take place in environments that are stress-free, calm and without distractions. The television should be turned off, noise and activity levels should be reduced and the person should be given undivided attention.

6

Therapeutic Interventions

This chapter explores the ways in which the social and psychological environment can be used to counteract some of the disabling impact of dementia. It will also identify interventions that support people in a way that builds on their strengths and minimises the potential threats to the person's coping abilities caused by inappropriate interventions.

The onset of dementia means that staff have to focus on maintaining skills, abilities and interests. This can present difficulties for staff, who have often chosen to work within the learning disability service because they want to enable people to grow and develop their full potential. They have often focused their involvement on finding new activities and challenges for the people who they support. If staff have been involved in this work, they can find it very disheartening to see those skills, which they have been instrumental in developing, starting to disappear.

It is important, however, to recognise that, despite the changes and losses that ensue from the onset of the dementia, there are many interventions that will help to maintain skills for as long as possible. They will also, of course, help to maintain a better quality of life.

People with dementia need to be helped to relax. Stress must be removed from their lives and positively relaxing interventions should be introduced. Simply sitting with their feet in a foot spa or having a beauty treatment such as a manicure or pedicure will provide relaxation. Having a cup of tea and a chat provides a constructive but relaxing activity. It is important to emphasise that the busy multi-activity days that many people with a learning disability engage in become inappropriate once they have dementia. This does not mean that people do nothing, but that they are offered and encouraged to engage in activities that are failure free and relaxing, and help them to maintain skills and contact with others.

It is important to stress that the suggestions made in this chapter are only techniques and only as good as the person who uses them. No single approach is a panacea. These are simply some identified ways of working that will enhance the person's ability to cope and maintain their skills as well as diminishing some of the disabling consequences of inappropriate interventions.

These interventions need to be placed within the context of the declining skills and developing different realities of the person with dementia.

The interventions considered in this chapter are as follows:

- developing failure-free activities
- reminiscence work
- life story work
- music
- touch
- aromatherapy.

Developing failure-free activities

One of the consequences of the progression of the dementia is that people become less and less able to instigate meaningful activities. This does not mean that they do not want to engage in such activities; it is often simply that they have lost the ability to self-start. This can lead to boredom, apathy and agitation, which can, of course, lead to challenging behaviours. Never assume that because a person's skills are deteriorating they are incapable of enjoying activity.

There is evidence (Kovach and Henschel 1996; Teri and Logsdon, 1991) that if people with dementia are given meaningful activity this will help to maintain functional abilities. It will increase social involvement and provide feelings of success and will lead to improved mood and a reduction in challenging behaviours.

People with dementia live in the moment (Rainbow 2003). This requires that the activities are immediately accessible, achievable and pleasurable. The fact that two minutes after completing an activity the person may have forgotten doing it does not detract in any way from the importance of supporting the person to do the activity in the first place. Whilst they are doing it, they are having a positive experience. It will make the person feel good. The feeling will probably last after the memory of the activity has gone.

It is important to develop activities that suit the person's level of functioning. The activities must be failure free otherwise they will simply reinforce the feelings of lack of self-worth and disability. The activities should also be pleasurable.

People working within the learning disability service, and particularly those working within day services, often feel under pressure to engage people in lots of activities. The need to demonstrate the achievement of goals can lead to a pursuit of constant activity and change; very often as a consequence day services are places of much activity and noise. There is often an expectation that throughout the day people will move between activities and rooms; for someone with dementia this will not be failure free and may result in increased levels of confusion and disorientation. It can be appropriate for someone to redo an activity if this gives them pleasure. They may well have forgotten that they have already done it. They may also remember that they have done it and that it was pleasurable and failure free.

Reduction in activities may mean that the person needs to arrive later at the centre, when all the hubbub at the start of the day has passed, and they may also need to leave early before they get tired and over-stretched and perhaps feel the effects of 'sun downing' (for more information on this see Chapter 11 on the environment). When deciding on the types of activity to use, try to develop activities that use things the person used to do and enjoy and then break the task down into parts. Give them the parts that they can still manage.

Case study 7

Mark, a man in his late forties, had always enjoyed working in the woodworking workshop. He had great skills, which he used to produce parts for chairs. He took great pride in the finished articles. As his dementia progressed, the noise in the workshop became too much for him to cope with;

he became increasingly agitated and confused. He also lost the dexterity needed to do the woodwork. He did, however, want to feel part of the work and to be with his friends and familiar staff.

A quieter room next to the workshop was cleared out and Mark was able to spend time in there with one member of staff and two other men who had dementia. They dusted, polished and cleaned the various items produced in the workshop before they were packaged for distribution.

This activity lasted for only a fraction of the time that had previously been spent in the workshop but it did provide structure and a sense of purpose and contact with friends. It also contained aspects of the previous activity.

Failure-free activities can be provided through visual stimulation. Looking through magazines, catalogues and papers will be undemanding and if it is done with a staff member on a one-to-one basis it will often become a source of conversation or even storytelling. Sitting with someone and giving of your time to an individual can create a sense of safety, comfort and stimulation (Kerr and Wilson 2001).

Being able to sit and look outside is a valid failure-free activity. The person is watching changes and will be stimulated by what they see. The person needs to be on the ground floor where they can more easily see what is going on. It is of concern, for this reason amongst others, that, in homes for older people, people with dementia are sometimes placed upstairs where they are further removed from the activities outside

Reminiscence work

It used to be thought wrong to encourage or even collude with older people's desire to reminisce. Dwelling on things in the past was considered in some way pathological, a regression to a past life, a denial of the passage of time and the reality of organic impairment. The remembrance of things past has been seen as a cause of unhappiness and even depression. In fact, whilst undoubtedly reminiscence can lead to feelings of regret for the passing of the time and particularly the passing of good times it can also, and generally does, act as a stimulus for happy memories that have a positive affect on a person's sense of well-being and self-esteem. O'Leary and Barry (1998) found in their reminiscence work with older people that there was raised self-esteem as well as happiness, well-being and socialisation.

Reminiscing is a normal, healthy activity in which we all engage. From about the age of 10 children start to reminisce. They will do this often with a sense of importance and belonging. We continue to reminisce throughout our lives. Reminiscence is not therefore something peculiar to old age, although of course the older we are the more we have to reminisce about.

It is through our history that we know who we are and what has formed us. It gives us a sense of our place in the world and therefore our sense of identity (Kerr 1997). Goldsmith (1996, p. 92) comments that 'reminiscence work helps people to use the then and there of life to enrich the here and now'. In relation to people with dementia, reminiscence takes on an even more powerful role. As the present becomes more fragmented and increasingly inaccessible, the person can feel adrift in a world that does not make sense. Feelings of isolation and uselessness are a common and perhaps inevitable consequence. Memories of the past can become anchors to help steady and engage the person. The past memories help to explain and fill the present for people with dementia. This probably accounts for the fact that 'reminiscence therapy is one of the most popular psychosocial interventions in dementia care, and is highly rated by staff and participants' (Woods *et al.* 2006, p.1).

Most of the literature on and experience of reminiscence work has been in relation to older people in the general population. There is, however, some experience and literature on the use of reminiscence work with older people with a learning disability (Gibson 2006; Puyenbroeck and Maes 2002). There is much less experience in and literature on this area of work with older people with a learning disability and dementia. It is, however, an area that needs to be developed. I hope that the following will enable staff to start to develop this valuable area of work.

As people with a learning disability live increasingly long lives they also have a longer history to recall and share. For some people with a learning disability, the past may hold painful memories. Indeed for many people with a learning disability the past may well contain unexplained changes and losses as well as the experience of long-stay hospitalisation and institutionalisation. For these reasons two members of staff may need to be involved in any group reminiscence work. Nevertheless reminiscence handled appropriately is a positive experience and should be part of staff practice with people with a learning disability and dementia. It will inevitably be an aspect of person-centred planning but needs to be given conscious attention for people with dementia.

This is an activity that could very usefully be introduced into day services as an alternative to some of the more demanding group activities that require people to be clearly rooted in the here and now, when they would be more comfortable in the past. It can provide failure-free, person-centred, enjoyable experiences that enable people to talk about events for which they are more likely to have the vocabulary: old words remain as more recent ones fade.

Reminiscence work can be run as a group activity. For people with dementia the group often needs to be quite small. Two or three people will provide sufficient stimulation without being over-demanding. The group facilitator can use triggers such as old photos, pictures of old equipment, household items, toys, and videos of past events, music and even smells from the past. The provision of objects that can be used as they would have been in the past can be very enjoyable and stimulating for people who have lost the ability to communicate verbally: brass to be cleaned or washing with a washboard. This may not be something people did themselves, but they may well have watched their mothers or grandmothers do it. Finding out about people's past will give clues as to which objects will act as triggers. People are thus encouraged to talk about the memories that are recalled by these objects. These objects, which will be increasingly familiar to them as present-day objects, become alien and potentially frightening.

Setting up a reminiscence group

Careful thought needs to go into who is in the group. Try to find people who will have similar histories and likes. It is important before inviting people to a group to find out something about their personal history. This will enable workers to avoid painful areas and will also help to determine what themes and triggers would be useful for the group.

Identify themes around which reminiscence can be developed, for example:

- housework
- days out
- children's games
- transport
- shopping
- the seasons.

Staff need to develop ideas of their own but also where possible from the people who are attending the group.

The triggers for each theme need to cover various senses and abilities. Do not just rely on sight. Many people will have difficulty with their vision. The use of music can be a very powerful trigger to reminiscing and can lead to people sharing the same songs. Use of smell should also be encouraged. Our sense of smell generally declines with age, but the provision of different smells from the past can be highly evocative and stir many memories. The use of scents and soap smells and cleaning smells should be considered.

A difficulty often experienced is the accumulation of triggers to be used as memorabilia in reminiscence work. Museums can be a good source of materials: some will hire out boxes of objects. Relatives often have things to contribute that are particularly pertinent to the person with dementia. Useful and inexpensive material can be sourced from charity shops, car boots and jumble sales. The development of themed memory boxes can help to determine the type and range of materials required.

Within the scope of this book it is not possible to provide a thorough coverage of the various issues in relation to setting up reminiscence work. For staff who want to develop their knowledge and skills, the Age Exchange Reminiscence Centre in Blackheath, London, provides invaluable resource material, ideas and training (Osborn 1999). This recommendation is given with the proviso that their material is for older people within the general population and so some of their themes and triggers are inappropriate, but they do provide a starting point for staff to begin to develop their own reminiscence work.

For many people with a learning disability and dementia, the group activity may prove to be too stimulating. There may be difficulty following the various contributions and the noise level may be too high. It will be hard for them to feel in control of what is happening. In this case one-to-one work is much more appropriate. One-to-one reminiscence can be done using the same objects and stimuli used for group activities or by using more personal memorabilia. Visiting old familiar places can be a great trigger for reminiscence. This will also feed directly into life story work.

Life story work

Life story work is an intervention that involves the recording and sharing of a person's past. It is true to say of people with dementia 'if you do not know their past then you cannot understand their present' (Kerr and Wilkinson 2005). It is vital, therefore, that as much significant information as possible is gained and recorded about people's past lives.

The need to record the information is particularly important within the context of a service where there is a high staff turnover, which can lead to a loss of unrecorded information. Although many staff will have long-term relationships with people they support, there is no guarantee that they will still be working with the person in years to come when the person might develop dementia. The recording of life stories will enable staff to understand and care for the people they support in the present and in the future.

Critically, without the information there is a danger that, if the person develops dementia, staff and carers will misinterpret the changed behaviours of the person and respond inappropriately.

Case study 8

George is a man with Down's syndrome and a diagnosis of Alzheimer's type dementia. He is in his fifties and has lived in and been supported by a village community organisation since he was 10 years old.

George's passion was cars and had been ever since he was a boy. His interest in cars extended to getting in them as often as possible, being taken for drives and also, if he was agitated, using them as a source of relaxation.

George developed dementia. One day he came out on to the front step of his house. The car was waiting to take him on a trip. He froze. He refused to get into the car. He kept saying, 'No, no, no' and asked where Cameron was: 'Find Cameron, get Cameron.' He became agitated and distressed very quickly. An apparent stubbornness appeared that had not been seen before. So the trip was cancelled. The next day the same thing happened again.

Initial enquiries to try to find out who Cameron was proved useless. The possibility that there had been a staff member who once worked at the community was investigated but no one of that name appeared to have worked there or indeed had been known to George.

George's brother was contacted to give information for his life story work that had just been undertaken at the community. George's brother sent a photo album with photos of George when he lived at home up to the age of 10. The photos were of George, clearly living in some luxury, with his own horse. Many of the photographs were of him sitting in his car with his 'driver' called Cameron, who had been assigned to care for George. George had been told 'Always wait for Cameron, go nowhere without him'.

What this revealed was that George now believed that he was the 10-year-old child. Attempts by people to get him into a car led to his refusal because he was waiting for Cameron to arrive. Without the life story work being undertaken, the staff would not have guessed the significance of what George was saying and doing. George was not being 'stubborn' or 'awkward' and his behaviour was that of a 'good boy' doing as he had been told. The potential to interpret his behaviour as 'challenging' and to respond inappropriately is high when the meaning and motivation for the behaviour is not known.

This information also helped to explain George's lifelong interest in cars. Cars were associated with a time when he had had this man's undivided attention and care. They were a symbol of being cared for and of course getting out and about.

Life story work is important for many reasons other than the essential one of enabling carers and staff to understand the meanings behind changed behaviour. Life story work means that there is a record of the person's past. It provides information about all aspects of the person's life. It goes beyond the dementia and emphasises the whole person. People with dementia are at significant risk of losing their sense of self-esteem and identity (Cheston and Bender 1999). Life story work can help to maintain these aspects by focusing on the things the person did, things they were good at and enjoyed. It emphasises their personality through their past experiences and memories. It therefore provides a vehicle for focusing on the person. In this way it provides a basis for communication and so will facilitate an increase in interaction. This will help prevent the lack of sense of importance and self-worth that comes from reduced communication and interaction with others.

The consequence of increased interaction and expectations is evidenced in the finding that when someone moves to another setting the staff in the new setting will have higher expectations of the person with dementia if they have had life story work done and this is made available to staff. This means that they are less likely to be ignored and more likely to receive positive attention from staff who might otherwise not feel able to find any point of contact. This is clearly important in terms of maintaining communication and well-being for the person with dementia. It is also important in the light of the findings of research (Wilkinson *et al.* 2004) which found that people with a learning disability and dementia are often ignored when they go into older people's services or hospital. This not only impacts on their sense of well-being but also more crucially can lead to them not being washed, clothed or supported to eat well. The latter can result in unnecessary morbidity and even death. (This issue is covered in more detail in Chapter 16 on models of care.)

Likewise when new staff come into the person's life, life story work provides vital information and a focus for communication and relationship building. In organisations that depend on the use of bank or agency staff this should be given an even higher priority.

As dementia progresses it can be hard to find suitable activities that will not stress the person or set them up to fail. Life story work, so long as only positive memories are recorded, can provide a suitable failure-free activity. The focus on the past also encourages staff to attend to people's need to reminisce.

The involvement of relatives is an aspect of life story work that needs to be encouraged and is, indeed, encouraging. Relatives will have memories and possessions from the person's past. They, as with George's brother, will often have much information about them before they entered into the learning disability services. Carers are often surprised and delighted to realise that their shared history is so important.

As dementia progresses previous activities will become problematic for people. The need to develop stress- and failure-free activities should be the focus of activity-based interventions. The use of life story work that does not focus on past painful, unhappy experiences and memories fits the bill perfectly. The person is able to easily access objects and stories that have meaning and give pleasure.

Developing life story work

Developing life stories involves a series of activities that will probably result in the production of a book and/or a box of memorabilia, but this is not the focus of the work. It is important to see this as a work in progress and not focus on the end product. The process of talking to people about their memories and of collecting objects and pictures should be treated as an activity in its own right.

The use of a box of objects and stories can be very powerful. People with a learning disability and dementia may have difficulty turning pages: they may also not remember to turn a page. A box allows them to see things clearly. It also importantly means that objects that they like to touch are easily available. Objects from their past that hold important memories can more easily be accessed by them.

Be as imaginative as you can about the possible contents of the box. A woman whose mother had had dementia, so she knew what happened as the condition progressed, decided that she wanted to take a video camera to her day centre and to all her friends and relatives. She asked them to tell stories about her life. She stated clearly she wanted this in her life story box so that when her dementia progressed she could sit and listen to people telling the stories.

The use of important and well-known music from the person's past can be evocative and provide a source for reminiscence and stories (other chapters focus more fully on the role and use of music for people with dementia).

It is important to leave the work in an accessible place with the proviso that confidentiality and the protection of the contents are maintained. Remember also that the life story materials belong to the person and no one else has right of access.

This fact was underlined by a story box which had the following paragraph attached:

This is my life story box.

I don't mind you looking through the box at the 'memories' that make up my life as long as you ask permission first and also that you take care, as it is very special to me. I would like you to look at my life story work and talk with me about all the memories in it. Please remember that this box contains a lot of private and personal memories and should be treated with respect at all times. Thank you.

When developing life story work there will often be a conflict about what is true and what is not. The difference in recall between people involved in events can lead to staff seeking 'the truth'. Resist the pursuit of accuracy and record the person's own version of what happened and who was involved.

Possible barriers to developing life story work

Although there are a number of potential obstacles to doing life story work, especially with people with a learning disability, they are all surmountable. A frequently highlighted problem is the fact that many older people with a learning disability spent much of their life in long-stay hospitals. Many people came out of these hospitals with very little information about their lives.

I know of a man of whom the only comment when he left a long-stay hospital to live in the community was 'Eric has had an uneventful 30 years.' Whilst this is, undoubtedly, an extreme case, it is true that very little of the years that people spent in the hospital was recorded and passed on to the new providers of support. This lack of information can make developing life story work problematic, but this is all the more reason for undertaking the work.

People's lives are not uneventful. There were public as well as private events that need to be captured. Large institutions usually placed much emphasis on public events such as festivities: Christmas and Easter were usually well marked. These can be used as a starting point for exploring the events of people's lives.

A further expressed obstacle is a lack of time. Life story work can be perceived as yet another thing that staff have to do. Good practice, however, would dictate that staff should be listening and attending to the people they support. Life story work simply involves the recording of these stories. As a meaningful, enjoyable and failure-free activity it could be substituted for other activities that have become too demanding or perhaps meaningless for the person. Further, by recording the stories and dialogue the staff member indicates that they have valued what the person has told them.

Possible things to include in life story work

- good times
- stories from the past about anything that the person is interested in
- achievements
- important people now and in the past
- hobbies now and in the past
- places stayed
- holidays
- relationships
- favourite songs
- likes and dislikes
- hopes and wishes
- favourite sayings.

Use a life story box as well as a life story book. Include a variety of things, such as:

- pictures
- photos
- music tapes, CDs and records
- old programmes
- ornaments
- toys
- dolls and furry animals

- fabrics
- things that have special smells.

Good practice in life story work

Here are some suggestions on what to avoid doing:

- Don't feel that you need to record everything.
- Don't let pressure for accuracy overshadow the need to understand the underlying feelings and emotion.
- Don't see life story work as a task to be completed.
- Don't be constrained by thinking that photographs are the only way to illustrate a life story book.
- Don't see life story work as a separate activity: it feeds into other work such as reminiscence groups, outings and care planning.
- Don't leave the individual 'trapped' in the past after a session of life story work.

(Adapted from Murphy 1994))

Here are some suggestions for good practice in life story work:

- Tell the individual with dementia what you are proposing to do and ask for permission to do it.
- Think about what preconceptions you might bring to the situation, for example doubt rather than belief.
- Try to understand what it might feel like to have such information recorded.
- Be aware of the variety of ways in which life story work may be used: by staff, by family carers and by the person with dementia.
- See the life story work as an organic activity.
- Use triggers when doing life story work and be aware that all five senses have the potential to be stimulated.
- Offer an environment relatively free of distractions.
- Include current material as well as historical details on the individual with dementia.

- Leave the life story book or box in an accessible place, subject to the constraints of confidentiality.

- Remember who 'owns' the book.

- Acknowledge sadness and grief when these emotions are expressed.

(Adapted from Murphy 1994)

Music

Music engages us sensually and emotionally. It is also a way in which many people choose to relax and deal with stress. For those whose cognitive skills are deteriorating, the use of music can be at least as important and perhaps more significant in their experience of relaxation and pleasure.

Music can also be used to facilitate participation and engagement with others. The importance and retention of rhythm has been demonstrated in people with middle-stage dementia. Clair (1996) observed that participation with rhythm is sometimes spontaneous and seems almost automatic. She records that 'when people with severe dementia are handed a mallet, which they receive with their dominant hand, and then a drum, which they receive with their non-dominant hand, they often begin to play even without receiving a request to do so' (Clair 1996, p. 79). This playing will desist unless prompted by another. But if someone else plays, the person will restart.

What is so important about this observation is that amongst people who have perhaps lost their verbal skills, are no longer able to carry out activities of daily living and are becoming potentially isolated from others the use of rhythm in accompanied playing can re-engage them.

People who have lost many of their verbal skills will often sing entire songs. Singing makes no cognitive demands. The importance of accentuating the positive in dementia care would suggest that it is a missed opportunity not to encourage this retained skill.

The willingness of staff to sing along is important. To have someone singing with you gives a clear message that you are being listened to and that someone is 'in tune' with you. There is evidence (Clair 1996) that if carers sing to people with dementia this can have a positive affect on behaviour. Singing can be associated with positive experiences and people from the past. Many people will have been sung to as children. This singing will often have been at times of nurturing: feeding, bathing and cuddling.

The singing of songs of childhood and the use of background music (Gotell 2003) at times when intimate tasks are being performed has been shown to reduce levels of 'challenging behaviour', probably because of the association with past caring and love.

Ragnoskog (1994) found that people with dementia were 'less irritable, anxious and depressed and ate more when music was played during dinner'. All this suggests that the use of music not only provides pleasure but also is an intervention that supports and enables people in other areas of their daily living.

There is need, however, for a caution. I had been encouraging managers to use music to calm people they supported. It was later discovered that the music was left on all day. The staff were irritated and actually made tense by the constant presence of the music. Presumably it was having a similar effect on the people they supported, who were unable to turn the music off. A constant backdrop of music may simply add clutter to the environment and cause agitation. Clair (1996) emphasises the need to monitor the amount of music that is played. She suggests that to have the best stimulative effect music should be played on a schedule, generally for 15–20 minutes every hour.

Fast tempo music may increase energy levels but it will also increase agitation. If someone is agitated use calming music. This is particularly relevant when people are pacing or wandering in an agitated state.

It is important to remember that the music that people listen to and find familiar will change as their dementia progresses. In the early stages they may listen to a whole variety of music from many different stages of their life. As the condition progresses they will return to earlier and earlier musical memories. Prinsley (1986) noted that music memory tended to be fixed between the ages of 15 and 24. This would suggest that this is well-remembered music. Of course what this music is will vary from individual to individual. Many people with a learning disability may have been living with their parents in their twenties and their parents' taste might be what they heard at that time. Eventually people will return to the songs and tunes of childhood.

It may be advisable in the evenings to play melodies rather than songs. People sometimes wake in the night saying that they can hear the words of a song going round in their head (Kerr 1997). There are no single responses in the use of music. The only way to determine how, when and what to play is by carefully observing the person with dementia and adjusting the music accordingly.

Touch

The importance of touch as a form of and aid to communication has been referred to in the chapter on maintaining good communication. Here the emphasis is on the ways in which touch can enable and support people to relax, feel secure, be less agitated and reduce anxiety and fear.

Chapter 4 on different realities highlights the terrible sense of loss, grief, anxiety and even abandonment that the person with dementia can experience. All of us at such times need comfort, warmth and reassurance. This is most easily given through the appropriate use of touch.

Case study 9

Alexander, a 69-year-old man with a learning disability and dementia, would become very distressed as he got tired in the afternoon. This distress was increased if other tenants were making a noise or moving around with various activities. Alexander would start to make high-pitched screaming noises and shake his body. A few minutes sitting with a member of staff with his head on their shoulder in a big hug calmed him. He would smile at the staff member with pleasure and was clearly comforted and relaxed.

As the condition progresses, the need for touch will increase. In the late stages when people are unable to vocalise, cannot control their mobility and bodily functions and can appear to be isolated and alone, touch becomes a way of maintaining human contact and reassuring the person that they are not alone.

Clair (1996, p.85) comments that 'touching can include holding hands, hugging, holding and rocking, sitting in close proximity, placing an arm about the shoulder, gently stroking the brow or cheek, kissing and caressing the face. Gentle massage using skin-conditioning creams or oils'.

I use a video in training that shows support for people with a learning disability and dementia in the Netherlands. After the video has been shown, the first or at most second comment by the audience is about the amount of touching that is used. There may be an element of cultural influence. Maybe Dutch culture is more tactile, maybe not. It is of course true that different cultures have different attitudes to touch and the British culture may be less tactile than some. However, what is clear is that the person with dementia will have the same needs in any culture. Social niceties will be gone and basic human need is what must be responded to.

At the very least staff should consider using foot and hand massage as planned and recognised ways of providing touch. It is, however, sad to reflect that if policies are too restrictive this might be the only way that someone gets a fundamental human need met.

For people working with those with a learning disability there is a particular issue that needs to be addressed. Very often staff have been involved in helping the people they support to use touch appropriately. This has sometimes involved programmes to reduce the amount of hugging and kissing that the person has been giving. The need to learn to hug and kiss when appropriate will sometimes even be translated into 'you don't hug or kiss'. This will present problems when staff begin to hug and kiss the person with dementia. This is particularly problematic if these two responses exist alongside each other within the same house amongst a group of tenants or in a residential setting between residents. This underlines the need to help others with a learning disability understand the impact of dementia. (The importance and method of providing training and information for peers of the person with dementia is dealt with in Chapter 9 on the experiences and needs of peers.)

There is a need to recognise that touch can be abusive and inappropriate. This is a reason not to abandon it but to find ways to use it legitimately and without fear that affection and warm caregiving will be misinterpreted. It makes it imperative that staff are clear about the policy of their organisation on the use of touch. It is also imperative that the policy is well informed and enlightened.

Aromatherapy

Aromatherapy is the therapeutic use of essential oils derived from plants. The oils are generally used in one of three ways. They can be applied directly to the skin: in this case they are often accompanied by a massage. They can be heated in an oil burner to produce a scent or they can be placed in a bath. It is thought that one of the ways in which the oils work is through the volatile constituents in the essential oils exerting physiological effects that result from absorption though the skin and/or respiratory system (Buchbauer, Jirovitz and Jager 1993).

The beneficial effects gained from the use of aromatherapy have been demonstrated in a number of studies. One study, which analysed the effect of gentle hand treatment with three essential oils, found specific improvements in people with dementia. These improvements included increased alertness, self-hygiene, contentment, initiation of toileting, sleeping at night and reduced levels of agitation, withdrawal and wandering (Kilstoff and Chenoweth 1998). A study into the use of Melissa or lemon balm showed significant improvements in wandering, shouting and screaming. There was a significant reduction in the time people were socially withdrawn and a significant increase in the amount of time people were engaged in constructive activities (Ballard *et al.* 2002). One of the challenges when supporting people with dementia is to maintain appropriate levels of communication and stimulation. Smells can be evocative and stimulate memories, which can then encourage people to talk. This is particularly useful in early stage dementia. The use of aromatherapy with essential oils when combined with hand and foot massage provides a form of relaxation and legitimate touch. This intervention can be easily learned. Alternatively a qualified aromatherapist will be able to advise on the use of essential oils. It is important when using oils to seek advice if people are on medication as some oils will interact with certain drugs.

In some instances the use of oils can be a substitute for certain drugs. People with dementia, and especially people with more advanced dementia, tolerate neuroleptic medication poorly. These drugs are often used for the reduction of agitation, wandering, sleeplessness and challenging behaviour. They can, however, cause Parkinsonism, drowsiness and falls, accelerated cognitive decline and even increased mortality.

Burns *et al.* (2002) have suggested that aromatherapy may sometimes be a useful alternative to the use of neuroleptic drugs for people with dementia.

Summary

This chapter describes a number of ways in which people with dementia can be supported and enabled to engage in failure-free activities that will enhance their sense of well-being and help to maintain skills. The use of reminiscence work and the development of life story work capitalise on their increasing return and attachment to the past. Life story work also enables staff to know more about the person's history. This should help staff better understand new and sometimes challenging behaviours. The use of music, touch and aromatherapy will provide calming, sensitive and enjoyable activities that help to counteract the stresses and challenges that face the person with dementia.

7

Challenging Behaviour

People with a learning disability, for a variety of reasons, more often present with behaviour that challenges their carers and services than their non-disabled age-matched peers (Meyer and Evans, 1994). The consequent higher expectation of the existence of challenging behaviour amongst people with a learning disability is compounded when they develop dementia because there is a tendency to see challenging behaviour as an inevitable aspect of dementia (Stokes and Goudie 1990). It is crucial that staff and service providers recognise that challenging behaviour in people with dementia is not necessarily an inevitable consequence of the condition.

It is depressing to see people moved between providers and settings because of their 'challenging behaviour' when close analysis of the situation will often reveal that the behaviour is being caused not by the dementia or the disability but by an external factor that could and should be removed.

It is both disturbing and optimistic to note that 'only 2% of aggressive events (involving people with dementia) have been found to occur without an antecedent event' (Ryden, Bossenmaier and McLauchlan 1991) disturbing because it acknowledges the amount of 'challenging behaviour' that is induced by extrinsic factors but optimistic because it highlights the fact that staff, carers and building designers can directly influence the reduction in aggressive events by attending to their own behaviours, interactions and designs.

Information on the impact of design on behaviour is to be found in Chapter 11 on physical environments. In this chapter attention will be directed towards the ways in which the social, psychological and emotional environment of the person with dementia can prompt challeng-ing behaviour.

Consider the following: imagine that you are in your bed at home. The bedroom door opens and you see a stranger standing there. They come up to you. They take the bedclothes down and start to undress you. What would you do? It is fairly likely that you would do one or more of the fol-lowing:

- scream
- hit out
- fight back
- cling to your clothes
- bite the person
- kick
- try to run away.

All of these responses would be perceived as healthy and appropriate. If you had dementia, however, and had exactly the same experience (because you no longer recognise your carer) and responded in the same way, then your behaviour might be seen as aggressive, uncooperative and problematic, i.e. challenging (Kerr and Cunningham 2004).

Challenging behaviours usually take place during a personal care activity (Moniz-Cook, Woods and Gardener 2000). This is primarily because people with dementia have reduced cognitive skills and are at risk of misidentifying and misinterpreting the social, emotional and physical environment. This misidentification and misinterpretation can be, and often is, exacerbated by the level of noise that is present at the time of the interaction. People with dementia have a decreased ability to filter out unwanted noise (Jacques and Jackson 2000) and activity and this can lead to increased anxiety and agitation, which further impairs coping and comprehension.

The need to pay attention to the social and emotional environment is underlined by research findings that have found a significant reduction in the risk of challenging behaviour when the minimal intervention of smiling and remaining relaxed during personal care tasks is employed

(Burgener *et al.* 1992). Further findings indicate that if the carer sings, preferably childhood songs, during the performance of intimate tasks this again significantly reduces challenging behaviour (Gotell 2003).

The reduction of challenging behaviour does, however, involve more than just these particular interventions. The need to assess the situation fully and identify what needs to be put in place is a challenge to carers. To be successful the following need to be addressed:

- Discover what the trigger for the behaviour is.
- Understand the emotions behind the behaviour.
- Understand what the person is trying to communicate.
- Understand the meaning of the behaviour.
- Try to see the world from the perspective of the person with dementia.

(Kerr 1997)

Consider the following case study.

Case study 10

Michael is 49 years old. He has Down's syndrome and a diagnosis of Alzheimer's disease. He has lived in supported accommodation for five years after spending most of his life in a large institution. For the last few weeks he has become agitated most evenings around tea-time. He has started to push the person who is making a pot of tea. He pushes them and then grabs the pot. Recently the pot fell to the floor during the incident and smashed.

Once he has the pot, he makes the tea and then puts the kettle in the cupboard. If another tenant goes to the cupboard at this time, Michael verbally abuses them. However, it seems that the staff are allowed into the cupboard and they are allowed to touch the teapot without Michael being concerned. Once tea is over he becomes less agitated.

The explanation for Michael's behaviour is to be found in his past. When he was in long-stay hospital he had the responsibility for making the tea. If he failed to do so, staff scolded him. He was frightened that if someone else made the tea then he would be in serious trouble. It was an important job, it was his responsibility and it was one of the few times that he felt important. The making of tea seemed to act as a trigger, causing Michael to be reminded of his role in the making of tea. Because of his impaired memory the past event has now become a present role and places an imperative on him.

There is always a strong possibility when people with dementia exhibit challenging behaviour that we attribute it to present reality. It is important that we recognise that it may be a past reality that is giving meaning and motivation to the behaviour.

Using ABC charts

The use of ABC charts can provide a way to develop systematic data gathering. It will enable carers to record all the elements that interact to create a challenging situation. People who work with those with a learning disability may already be familiar with the use of the ABC chart as a process of identifying and understanding the causes of challenging behaviour. It is important that this process is continued for someone with dementia. The problem is that the behaviour being identified and its meaning and motivation may well be rooted in the person's part, a past that staff may not know about, especially if it is not recorded in life story work.

Most challenging situations involve a complex interaction of the person with dementia, the social and physical environment, their history and the personalities of all involved. How does ABC work? It is simply a way of organising information under the following headings:

- **A**ctivating event
  - Who was around at the time or just before the event?
  - When did the event occur?
  - Where did the behaviour occur?
  - What was the person doing immediately before the event?
  - What was happening at the time and just before the event?
- **B**ehaviour
  - Is this behaviour new?
  - What form did it take? Was it verbal or physical?
  - What words did the person use?
  - What or who was the target of the behaviour?

- ○ How long did it last?
- ○ Describe the behaviour precisely.
- • Consequences
  - ○ How did others respond to the event?
  - ○ Was the person told off, ignored, sedated or restrained?
  - ○ How did the person respond to the way others approached the event?

In relation to the section where behaviour is described, it is very important that what is recorded is clear, descriptive, concrete and objective. Describing someone's behaviour as 'aggressive' is not good enough. What one person considers aggressive another may consider an acceptable form of communication. To understand the meaning and motivation of behaviour it is often necessary to pick up on the nuances of what is said and done.

Consider the situation where a member of staff records that the women she supports has become 'very aggressive at meal times'. On further enquiry it transpired that this aggression involved her throwing her food. This is a specific behaviour. The next questions to ask are 'Where did she throw her food?' and 'When did she throw her food?' If she threw the food on the floor, this may indicate that she was trying to communicate that she did not like or want the food. If she threw the food at the staff member then this might indicate that she did not like the staff member or did not like the way she was feeding her. The response to one action might be to change the food; the response to the other would be to change the staff member or to get her to change the way she was helping the person to eat.

The information often needs to be recorded over a three-week period to allow for staff changes, weekends, changes in routines and other occurrences that might not happen every day or every week.

An ABC chart will facilitate the keeping of organised, regular information (see Figure 7.1).

Remember to consider the following common possibilities as explanations of challenging behaviour:

- • Is there too much activity?
- • Is there too much noise?

- Is the person in pain?
- Is the person bored?
- Is the person tired?
- Has something frightened them?
- Are they confused and trying to do something from their past which they are being prevented from doing?

Date	A	B	C	Comments

Figure 7.1 An ABC chart

Personal responses to behaviour

It is important that staff are aware of their own responses to challenging behaviour. It is easy, through our reactions, to exacerbate the situation. The following do's and don'ts will enable staff to better de-escalate and calm the situation.

- Stay calm.
- Avoid invading the person's space.
- Touch the person gently if possible, but make sure they see you first.
- Use gentle calming music.
- Turn off any music that has an insistent or agitating beat.
- Give plenty of room.
- Reassure no harm will come.
- Listen, and encourage talk rather than action.

- Remove any audience, when and if possible.
- When possible divert attention.
- Don't confront the person.
- Avoid shouting or raising your voice.
- Don't touch or move in a manner indicating an attempt to control.
- Don't move rapidly, especially from behind.
- Don't tease, ridicule or restrain.
- Don't show fear, alarm or anxiety.
- Avoid cornering the person.

Adrenalin stays in the body up to 90 minutes after arousal. This means that even though things might seem to have calmed down, everyone involved in the situation is still primed to react more quickly to any new threat or misunderstanding. This means that attention needs to be paid to keeping the environment calm and to reassuring the person with dementia.

The list and comments above are easy to write but not always easy to do. Staff need help, support and training if they are going to be enabled to manage such situations.

The need to walk and 'wander'

Wandering is something that we all engage in. It is a normal and natural behaviour that gives pleasure and healthy activity. We talk about it and poets write about it. Wordsworth 'wandered lonely as a cloud' and yet when someone with dementia walks about and wanders this is often perceived as an inevitable problem and a form of 'challenging' behaviour.

This 'challenging behaviour' is being considered separately because it is particularly characteristic of people with dementia and because unlike other challenging behaviours it is one that, to a considerable extent, we should be encouraging or at least supporting. Unfortunately, however, not only is it a behaviour that is often discouraged but also it can result in people being moved unnecessarily to new and often 'secure' accommodation.

The concerns held by staff about people 'wandering' are understandable and are supported by findings that indicate that nearly 25 per cent of people in care who 'wander' experience a fatal or serious injury (Kiely, Morris and Algase 2000). This underlines the importance of the need to be proactive in setting up situations and opportunities that will enable people to walk about safely. If staff do not take this more positive and encouraging approach they may place the person with a learning disability and dementia at risk of serious injury or sedentary boredom.

Case study 11

Jack, a man in his seventies with a learning disability and a diagnosis of dementia, used to work in a hotel as a night worker. He had the job of collecting shoes from outside bedrooms and cleaning them during the night. Jack had given this job up many years before the onset of the dementia. Recently when the other residents in his home went to bed, Jack set off with great agitation down the road.

Staff initially saw this as 'wandering' behaviour. Most of the staff did not know about his previous job; when this was revealed it became clear that the trigger for this behaviour was the coming of darkness and people going to bed. To try to stop Jack would lead to him becoming agitated and even abusive. In his mind he was going to be late for work. He was not 'wandering', he was doing something purposeful. Without the background information it may well have been that he was seen as developing challenging, wandering behaviour.

The staff had two options. Jack clearly needed to leave for work. One solution was for staff to set off down the road with him. He soon forgot the trigger that had set him off and he would return with staff after a few minutes. The staff later placed shoes outside other residents' doors and Jack was happy to engage in his role as collector and cleaner of shoes. After a while staff announced to him that the job was done and he could now go to bed himself.

This case study illustrates the way in which the trigger for the behaviour may be linked to past events or situations that may be unknown to the carer.

Case study 12

Margaret was 56 years old and had Down's syndrome and dementia. The staff at her day service were increasingly anxious about her increased 'wandering'. She had been found on a number of occasions 'wandering' around outside the day centre.

On investigation it transpired that she had set off to go to the toilet. She had failed to locate this but had seen the fire door. Seeing the way out amply visible though the glass of the fire door and having forgotten why she had set off, Margaret left the building. She was now engaged in a completely different activity, walking around the garden, a habit she had pursued extensively when she lived in a long-stay hospital.

(See Chapter 11 on the environment for advice on dealing with the issue of fire doors.)

What these case studies illustrate is that what can appear as aimless wandering will usually have a logical and clear explanation. The problem for staff and the person with dementia is that the person with dementia may forget what triggered the behaviour or they may not be able to explain what it is they are trying to do.

There are many reasons why people wander when they have dementia. Most of them are exactly the same as the reasons why any of us wander and walk about. The difference is that the person with dementia may not be able to explain to us why they are doing it or where they are going. They may also have forgotten what they set off to do and they may be lost.

When trying to determine why someone is wandering or walking about, it is useful to consider the following possible explanations:

- *Physical discomfort:* the person may be walking about because they are trying to relieve the pain of constipation or arthritis.

- *Lack of activity:* if the person has been sitting doing little for a long period, they may simply be getting up and walking around for exercise.

- *Boredom:* if there is insufficient stimulation in the environment the person may seek stimulation for themselves. Walking about through new places will provide this. Simply being outside will provide new stimulation. It is important to continue with this even if the person themselves is no longer able to walk. The use of wheelchairs should be encouraged.

- *Separation anxiety:* there may be an anxiety about losing someone. The short-term memory loss means that the person may forget how long the other person has gone for. They may also have forgotten the promise that the person will return.

- *Searching:* this can occur when the person is looking for someone or a place that is lost to them. This activity is of course a normal part of grieving. The onset of dementia may return the person to the time of their loss and reactivate this grieving behaviour.

- *Reactivated previous behaviours:* triggers in the environment may connect with previous activities. These may serve to convince the person that they are now back at that stage of their life and there is an imperative for them to re-engage with the associated activity. The activation of past commitments that are well learned and had special meaning will often occur. Things such as work commitments, day centre attendance and other routines that are well embedded in the long-term memory may well trigger wandering behaviour.

- *Night-time wandering:* this is more likely to occur because of the reduction in information within the environment. The lack of light and the lack of other people will increase disorientation and may lead to the person wandering about trying to find something or someone familiar to them.

- *Apparent aimlessness:* the person may set off with a clear intention to go somewhere or do something but they may forget after a short time what the activity was that they sought to engage in.

It is important to determine the meaning behind and motivation for the wandering behaviour. If it is the result of agitation, pain and distress then these causes can be addressed and either prevented or eliminated. It may be, however, that the need to walk around should be aided and encouraged but with the proviso that a risk assessment is done and the activity can be supported with minimal risk. There is a paradox that, on the one hand, staff and carers are often at a loss to find suitable activities for people with a learning disability and dementia and yet, on the other hand, one activity that will stimulate and provide healthy activity is often seen as a 'challenging behaviour', so elicits a negative response and is often, as a consequence, discouraged.

One way to encourage wandering is, of course, through the provision of opportunities to walk about. Gardens and paths are an excellent way to deal with this issue. Ideally staff would also go out with people for walks or encourage others such as families, when they visit, to go for a walk. Too often relatives feel confined to the premises and can pick up on staff fears of their family member's 'wandering' behaviour.

Night-time disturbance

Case study 13

Charlie is a 52-year-old man with a diagnosis of dementia. He lives in a small residential provision for ten people. Charlie has started to wake at night. The first time that staff were aware of his waking was one night when he was found in the kitchen at 3 a.m. He was partly dressed and was trying to make some breakfast. He was in an agitated state and clearly worried that he was going to be late for the bus that took him to his day service. The staff member tried to explain to Charlie that it was 3 in the morning. He reinforced this by pointing at the clock. The clock had been moved to 7 o' clock. Charlie had moved the hands. He knew it was the morning so the clock was wrong and needed changing.

At other times Charlie would wake and shout out to others to get up. He would even bang on their doors. By the time the sleepover staff were awake, so were the other residents, who were starting to lose patience with Charlie's nocturnal disturbances. Attempts to get Charlie back to bed usually led to an increase in his agitation. He would shout and protest. If he did go back to bed promptly he would return to the kitchen within a short time and the process would start again. There was increasing concern that Charlie would no longer be able to stay in the present accommodation unless he was given sedation.

Night-time waking and disturbance caused by people with dementia can lead to high levels of stress and anxiety amongst staff and other tenants and residents as well as the person with dementia. Failure to deal with this issue can often lead to people being moved to other accommodation and/or being given night-time sedation when this could be avoided.

It is a frequent consequence of ageing that people will wake more often during the night. This is normal and natural. It should not be seen as pathological and unless it causes the person distress, it should be managed and supported.

The onset of dementia adds to the night waking and contributes complicating factors. People with dementia wake at night. This is partly the result of damage to the circadian rhythm, which is responsible for the brain knowing when it is day and night. The rhythm tells us when to get up and when to go to bed. Once the part of the brain that has this function is damaged, people with dementia will not be able to tell night from day.

It is common for people to wake at night and mistakenly think it is the morning. This will cause them to start to prepare for the day: they may get dressed, try to prepare breakfast and try to leave the premises. People will often be agitated, thinking that they are going to miss the bus and be late for their day service or worry that they will be late for work. This occurs because once they have woken they do not receive the message that if it is dark, the clock says 3 a.m. and no one else is about, they should return to bed. The message is 'I have woken up' and it is time to get up.

This can present staff with difficulties, as often the explanations about the time of night are not believed. The person will often be agitated and worried and they will interpret this feeling as the consequence of the need to get going, to do something, to achieve the morning routine. The temptation for staff in these circumstances is to try to get people back to bed too quickly. This can be counterproductive. The approach taken should be focused on reducing anxiety and disorientation. Spending time talking to the person, giving them a hot drink and something to eat, perhaps a hand massage and generally not rushing or contradicting them is the best approach. Once the person has relaxed then bed can again be suggested.

It is worth considering the fact that night-time waking may, far from being a nuisance, actually provide an opportunity. Wilkinson *et al.* (2004) found examples of night-time staff using the fact that someone was awake at night as an opportunity to give them one-to-one attention and also to provide a nutritious meal. This book has emphasised the need for people with dementia to have calm, failure-free environments with one-to-one support. It may be that such an environment exists more at 3 or 4 o'clock in the morning than at 3 or 4 o'clock in the afternoon.

This type of response does require the use of waking night staff. Wilkinson *et al.* (2004) found that the use of waking night staff rather than sleepover staff had a significant impact on the way in which night-time waking was dealt with. It had an impact not only for the person with dementia but also for other people living with them

If staff are awake then they can anticipate any disturbance; they can support the person and prevent some of the noise and movement that may wake others. They can provide activity and attention that reduces agitation and can spend time with the person until they return to sleep. The use of reclining beds in the sitting area can enable the person with dementia to remain close to staff. This can provide comfort and reassurance.

It is important that the sleep disturbance is not attributed uncritically to the dementia. Other causes such as the possibility that the person may be in pain, that they need the toilet or that the environment is noisy or too bright should be considered.

Staff should make sure that they do not talk too loudly, that they do not have the radio or television on and that doors do not bang and floors creak. The use of ringing alarms should be avoided. Staff need to have buzzers or flashing light alarms. Staff should also be wary of carrying out housekeeping activities that may make a noise. The use of the washing machine and dishwasher can significantly add noise during the night. This is not only from the machines themselves but also from the plumbing as the water supply is turned on and off.

Make sure that there are blackout curtains. An outside light can become a source of disturbance if it is allowed to shine into the bedroom. The message can be that it is light outside and so time to get up.

The significance of environmental cues in managing night-time disturbance was highlighted by members of one staff group, who realised that when the man they supported got up at night he saw them in their day clothes. Their clothing clearly gave a message that they were working and he interpreted this as a need for him to get dressed as well. The staff had nightclothes readily available to put on when the man got up. He took the cue from their attire and would return to bed.

As with all problematic behaviours there must be a systematic record of the time, nature and trigger. This information should inform decisions

NYACK COLLEGE MANHATTAN

about the best response. This may be to use medication but this should be used only after other avenues have been pursued. A sleep diary, taken from *Down's Syndrome and Dementia: Workbook for Staff* (Dodd, Kerr and Fern 2006, p. 51), should be kept for a period of at least one week (see Figure 7.2).

If sedation is given this must be monitored regularly and stopped as soon as reasonably possible. Night-time can be a time of anxiety and distress for everyone. The dark and isolation can be depressing and disturbing. It is a time when people will worry. The worries that in the day seem small can take on mammoth proportions in the still of the night. This is no different for people with dementia except inasmuch as they may feel

Day, date, time	What happened?	What did you do?	Outcome

Figure 7.2 A sleep diary

(Dodd, Kerr and Fern 2006)

even more isolated and alone and less able to think through their worries. Staff need to respond to these feelings rather than concentrate on the need to get people back to bed.

The use of medication

If after an assessment there appears to be no obvious environmental trigger or if the trigger identified is not one that can be removed then it may be necessary to use medication. This should be undertaken only when all other possible avenues have been explored and in the knowledge that many behavioural problems are of short duration.

Medication does have a role in the management of challenging behaviour amongst people with dementia, but it should never 'be commenced without a careful appraisal of the person's whole situation and the likely balance between overall benefit and adversity to the individual' (Hopker 1999, p. 108).

For further information on the use of medication for people with dementia, see Chapter 15 on issues in relation to medication.

Summary

It is crucial that staff and service providers recognise that challenging behaviour in people with dementia is not necessarily an inevitable consequence of the condition. Most challenging behaviours seen in people with dementia are triggered by the physical environment or by interactions with carers. This is something that staff and providers of care can do something about. The determination of the triggers to the behaviour can be facilitated by the use of the ABC chart. Once the trigger for the behaviour has been identified it is essential that all staff are aware of what it is and change their behaviour and/or the environment accordingly.

Wandering or walking about is usually a normal healthy activity. It is a behaviour that should often be encouraged rather than discouraged. It is important to determine, as with all behaviours, what the trigger for the behaviour is and, if possible, if it is a worthwhile thing for the person to do; then ways and means should be found to support them in this activity. If the walking about is causing problems then alternative responses are needed. These may include the use of medication.

People with dementia tend to wake at night; they are also likely to be disorientated in time and space. This can be disturbing not only for them but also for other residents and tenants. This is often the trigger for moving people to another setting. It is important to determine if there are any triggers to the waking that can be removed. It is often counterproductive if staff try to get people back to bed quickly. This is more likely to be the case where staff are employed in a sleepover capacity. The employment of waking night staff is essential. By the time the sleepover staff have woken, then so have the other people in the house. The use of waking night staff not only reduces disturbance to others, but also will help to reduce the agitation often experienced by the person with dementia. The night waking can be used in a positive way to give the person with dementia time on a one-to-one basis and also to provide them with the opportunity to eat in a calm environment.

If there do not appear to be any changeable triggers for the behaviour and if the person is distressed, then the use of medication will often be necessary. This should be used with caution, with the recognition that dementia is a progressive condition which means that the cause of the behaviour may disappear thus enabling the drug to be withdrawn.

Responding to the Pain Needs of People with a Learning Disability and Dementia

As people get older they are more likely to experience chronic pain. Tsai and Chang (2004) found that amongst older people in the general population 64–6 per cent experienced chronic pain. People with dementia are no less susceptible to pain and yet they are prescribed and given less pain relief than people without dementia (Horgas and Tsai 1998). So there is a high level of unrecognised and, therefore, untreated pain amongst people with dementia in the general population (McClean 2000).

Kerr *et al.* (2006) found that the pain experiences and pain management of people with a learning disability who have dementia mirrored findings in relation to people in the general population. Extra and compounding issues in relation to people with a learning disability were also identified.

The factors, which contributed to poor pain recognition and therefore poor treatment, were as follows:

- 'diagnostic overshadowing': attributing all changes to the impact of dementia
- the use of 'as required' medication
- communication difficulties associated with dementia
- previous history influencing present assessments
- beliefs about pain thresholds

- a focus within the service on behaviour that challenges
- professional awareness of the impact of older age on people with a learning disability.

Diagnostic overshadowing

Diagnostic overshadowing occurs when a diagnosis for one illness or condition becomes the explanation for all subsequent changes in the person's health and behaviour. There is evidence that the fact that someone has a learning disability can often 'override and obscure physical illness' (Ng and Li 2003, p.12). It is also recognised that within the general population of people with dementia there is a tendency to attribute changes in the individual to the progression of their dementia, rather than other causes (Mason and Scior 2004). Wilkinson *et al.* (2004) found that people with both a learning disability and dementia experienced the impact of these responses leading to 'diagnostic overshadowing'.

This is illustrated well in relation to explanations given for night-time disturbance amongst people with a learning disability and dementia. People with dementia wake at night (some reasons for this are suggested in Chapter 7 on challenging behaviour). There is, as a result, a tendency amongst those supporting people with dementia to attribute all night-time disturbances to the impact of the dementia. It is evident, however, that there are many non-dementia-related reasons why someone may wake at night. The existence of painful conditions is one of these.

One of the painful conditions that many people with a learning disability and dementia will experience is arthritis. This is a condition that is particularly painful at night when joints stiffen. Kerr *et al.* (2006, p. 26) recorded people's own descriptions of waking at night with arthritic pain: 'Well it [knee] swells if maybe I'm lying in bed sleeping and I wake up stiff' (woman with dementia), also 'Can't lie on that [hip], feel it in bed' (women with dementia). In both these cases staff were not picking up on the arthritis but were attributing night waking solely to the fact that the people had dementia. They were not offering any pain relief.

A focus within the service on behaviour that challenges

As described in Chapter 7 on challenging behaviour, people with a learning difficulty, for a variety of reasons, more often present with behaviour that challenges their carers and services than their non-disabled age-matched peers (Meyer and Evans 1994). Indeed 'challenging behaviour' is often given high priority on training courses for staff working with people with a learning disability. While this is a vital aspect of staff learning and skill development, it can lead to staff wrongly attributing challenging behaviours to other causes rather than pain, particularly when people with a learning difficulty develop dementia. If someone already has a history of behaviour that others find challenging, it is possible that when they exhibit that behaviour it is seen and understood as a repeat of previous behaviour rather than a new behaviour triggered by pain.

Pain is positively associated with screaming, aggression and verbal agitation in dementia (Cohen-Mansfield, Werner and Marx 1990). It is interesting to reflect on the types of behaviours that can result from pain experiences. Questionnaires to groups of staff about their responses to pain elicit most of the following:

- increased irritation
- moaning
- withdrawal
- crying
- screaming
- swearing
- aggression
- poor eating
- anxiety
- hitting out if touched or threatened to be touched in the painful area.

Many of these behaviours are also labelled as challenging amongst people with a learning disability who have dementia.

The following case study provides a good example of the way in which pain-related behaviour might be misinterpreted; it is taken from a study carried out by Kerr *et al.* (2006, p. 39; reproduced by permission of the Joseph Rowntree Foundation).

Case study 14

Jane is 51 years old. She has Down's syndrome and has been diagnosed with dementia. Every morning Jane screamed, shouted abuse and hit out as staff helped her out of bed and along to the bathroom. There was some feeling that this behaviour was because she did not want to get out of bed and face the day. She was seen as 'being stubborn'. This seemed to be confirmed by the fact that the screaming and hitting stopped after the bathing was done and as the day progressed. The morning procedure became increasingly distressing for everyone concerned.

Jane had arthritis: this is a painful condition that is worse in the mornings after the person stiffens up during the night. A decision was made to give Jane paracetamol 20 minutes before she got out of bed. This resulted in a complete change in her behaviour. She was clearly no longer in pain and went happily to the bathroom.

This case is an example of an alternative response to 'challenging behaviour'. Give pain relief and see if the behaviour changes. This is such a simple and obvious response that it is strange that it is not used more often. There is the possibility that if the giving of the drug is not recorded then another member of staff may repeat the dose. This is an issue about recording medications, not about the giving of pain relief. The giving of two paracetamol is not going to do harm but may provide vital relief. If it does then the person's behaviour will change and this will be an indication that the behaviour is caused by pain. The next stage is to identify where the pain is and what is causing it. The use of pain relief can, however, begin the process of proper diagnosis.

Communication difficulties associated with dementia

Pain is a highly subjective experience. Many things will influence how an individual will experience pain; culture, age, ethnicity and gender are the main variables. The person with pain is the only person who knows how severe and enduring the pain is. Others have to ascertain the nature of the pain through observation and communication. The need to pay attention to subtle and often almost imperceptible changes is critical. The awareness of the look of 'worried eyes' may be the key to pain recognition. Staff may already be attending to these changes in people they support. What is important is that when the person has dementia the same attention continues to be given to these observations.

One useful definition of pain is that 'pain is whatever the patient says it is, and occurs whenever the patient says it does' (McCaffery 1968, p. 95). Clearly this presents problems for pain identification in relation to people with dementia where communication is an increasing problem.

Many people with a learning disability will have experienced communication problems prior to the onset of dementia; often strategies have been developed to maximise the person's ability to communicate. With the onset of dementia these strategies begin to fail and communication deteriorates from the previously achieved level.

People will start to lose the words they might have had to describe pain. As described in Chapter 2, 'What is dementia?', damage to the parietal lobes results in a number of significant problems for pain communication. Amongst other things the left side parietal lobe is responsible for our understanding of patterns, essential for the use of language where the patterning of words is critical to communication. The left side lobe is also responsible for our understanding of the patterns and geography of our body: it tells us which is our right, which is our left side. Once the part of the brain that tells the person where their head, their foot, their left and their right are becomes damaged then they can no longer physically indicate where the pain is located. The person with a toothache not only might fail to find the word 'toothache', but also might be unable to locate the place where the pain is and will not be able to put their hand there.

People will sometimes use a general phase such as 'My head hurts' because they cannot find the word 'toothache', but they are communicating that there is a pain. This can lead to problems for assessment. If a person persistently says their leg hurts and yet they are walking well, there is a temptation to think that there is no pain and that the person wants attention. It may be that the pain is elsewhere.

People will often use phrases they used in the past as a generalised way of expressing pain. For example, people may constantly say they have a 'tummy ache' because this was a pain they would have had in their childhood and probably the one they best remember. This does not mean that this is the location of the pain; it is simply the use of a well-remembered pain-related phrase.

The person may use a phrase as a substitute for the correct word. 'Oh dear, oh dear' will indicate distress but there may be a failure to recognise this as an expression of physical rather than emotional pain.

Sometimes the communication will be not through words but through actions. The need to understand these is illustrated well by the following example given in the study carried out by Kerr *et al.* (2006, p. 22; reproduced by permission of the Joseph Rowntree Foundation).

Case study 15

Geoffrey is a 48-year-old man with Down's syndrome and dementia. He had lost all his teeth many years ago and had ever since worn dentures successfully without any complaint. After the onset of dementia he started to take his dentures out and would try to hide them. Staff kept giving them back and, with instructions from the most senior worker, insisted that Geoffrey wear them. He would again take them out and try to hide them. This went on for some time, with Geoffrey becoming more and more distressed at meal times when there was insistence on him wearing the dentures. No attempt was made to investigate his gums or to find out the meaning behind the changed behaviour.

One day his dentures had completely disappeared. In conversation a student working in the house commented that she had seen, to her amazement, Geoffrey up at the top of a tall tree in the garden. An investigation of the treetop revealed Geoffrey's dentures. Clearly Geoffrey had been trying to communicate, but in the end took things into his own hands and placed the dentures as far away as he possibly could.

An investigation of his mouth revealed painful gum disease.

Another interpretation of Geoffrey's behaviour might have been that, because of the dementia, his reality is that he is younger and at a time in his life when he did not wear dentures. He takes them out, as he does not understand why they are there. Events proved, however, that it is vitally important to consider pain as an explanation rather than automatically assuming he was being awkward and that the behaviour is related to the dementia.

Previous history influencing present assessments

Previously known behaviour patterns often influence assessments. If someone has in the past presented with certain behaviours, it is possible that the new behaviours will be seen as a regression to previous patterns. This may be the case but it might also be that the present behaviour, whilst similar to previous behaviours, now has a different cause and meaning. An example of this would be the man who was always a bit cantankerous and uncooperative. This was his personality and way of coping. The onset of gum disease after his diagnosis of dementia made him extremely bad tempered but this was not an extension of previous behaviour, although staff interpreted it as just 'him up to his old ways'.

It is important to remember that if we do not understand what is motivating behaviour then our assessment may be inaccurate. The motivation and meaning will change often with the onset of dementia and this might mask the fact that pain is now the underlying motivation for behaviours that previously would have been triggered by something else.

Beliefs about pain thresholds

There is a belief, which still persists, that people with a learning disability have high pain thresholds. People with a learning disability, like their non-disabled peers, will have individual and differing responses to pain. If some of these differences are exaggerated and generalised into a belief about pain thresholds, then there is a danger that there will be a reduced sensitivity amongst staff to the possibility that someone might be in pain.

It is important to recognise that past experiences may lead people to deny the existence of pain. Some older people with a learning disability may have experience of living in large institutions. Their experiences of staff responses to their pain will not necessarily be positive. I heard of a man who had had a toothache when he was 14 years old and had all his teeth taken out. This is both appalling and illustrative of good reasons why people might have learned to keep quiet about their pain. Less dramatically but still a determinant of people's reaction to pain is the recognition that in large institutions people did not necessarily get the attention they needed. People's pain was often ignored. Staff were overworked and did not necessarily have the time for the type of attention people required. If someone has learned not to complain early in their life then this is the behaviour that they will return to when they develop dementia.

The use of 'as required' medication

Pain relief is often prescribed 'as required'. This is problematic in relation to people with dementia. If, as indicated, people supporting the person with dementia do not know when the person is in pain, then how can they be certain that they know when it is 'required'. There is evidence within the general population that for people with dementia not only is there less prescribing of analgesia than amongst an age-matched population without dementia, but also even when analgesia is prescribed to a person with dementia, 83 per cent did not receive it (Dawson 1998).

For these reasons the prescribing of analgesia 'as required' is not recommended for people with dementia. The World Health Organization (WHO 1996) guidelines on prescribing analgesia to people with dementia are clear. 'As required' should not be the primary approach to pain management for people with dementia. There should be regular administration; the treatment should be adjusted from one step to the next according to increasing or decreasing pain severity, history of response and side-effect profile (WHO 1996).

It is important that once analgesia is given there is a monitoring process. Because of the nature of the support that people with a learning disability receive a number of people may be involved in their care. Often a member of staff, carer or support worker may give pain relief and then by the time the effects have worn off someone else may be with the person. It is critical that all involved know about the pain relief given and that this is constantly evaluated. There may be a tendency amongst some people who have a reluctance to use drugs to under treat. This is not an option if the pain relief is going to be properly administered and monitored.

Professional awareness of the impact of older age on people with a learning disability.

Previously many people with a learning disability did not live into their old age. Education and training of those who work with and support people with a learning disability reflected this and so inevitably concentrated on the needs of younger people. This means that people are often ill-equipped with the necessary knowledge skills and indeed experiences to give informed responses to older people with a learning disability.

Kerr *et al.* (2006) found amongst the various groups of staff who supported and managed services for older people with a learning disability that the lack of awareness of the conditions of older age meant that they were, perhaps inevitably, unaware of the potentially painful conditions, such as arthritis, that people might be experiencing. This lack of experience and knowledge among professionals has an impact on the detection and management of pain in older people with a learning disability and dementia.

People will, of course, also experience painful conditions that are nothing to do with age but are particular to individuals as a result of their lifestyles, life events and individual health. It is significant then that even conditions that people have had for many years can be overlooked in old age. As in the general population, there is a danger that there is an acceptance of pain as an inevitable part of older age. This must be challenged.

Non-pharmacological interventions to relieve pain

Non-pharmaceutical interventions can prevent, reduce and relieve pain. For chronic musculoskeletal pain which is associated with increased age, the 'application of heat and massage or positioning can sometimes be all that is needed' (McClean 2003, p. 482). Chronic degenerative joint disease causes pain in the back and limbs; ostoeporotic spinal deformity also causes back pain. The need to support people's bodies with appropriate seating, the use of aromatherapy, massage and music to relax people and the slowing down of activities and interventions will all contribute to pain reduction.

People in pain will tense up and stiffen their body. The significance of almost all the above interventions is that they are directly or indirectly relaxing. They do not necessarily take the pain away but they may make the secondary impact less and so may make it more tolerable. The use of some of these interventions at night, especially aromatherapy, would help people to sleep better. The use of individually adapted chairs is important. These may well serve to reduce the occurrence of pain as well as giving support and comfort to parts of the body that are painful.

A number of these interventions involve touch. People with dementia need touching, both as a form of communication and as a source of comfort (Goldsmith 1996). People in pain are, as evidenced above, relieved of pain or at least enabled to cope with it through the appropriate use of touch.

Many of these interventions should already be part of the repertoire of support and help used with people with a learning disability. The important thing to note is that these need to be extended consciously to the use of pain prevention, reduction and relief, particularly when dementia is also present.

Summary

This chapter has identified that older people with a learning disability and dementia may, like the general population with dementia, be experiencing high levels of unrecognised and untreated pain.

This may be the effects of 'diagnostic overshadowing', the focus within the service on 'challenging behaviour' and the problems with communication that develop with the onset of dementia. The effect is compounded by a low level but still persistent belief that people with a learning disability have higher pain thresholds than other people. The detection of pain is further inhibited by reduced awareness amongst staff of the painful conditions of older age. The use of 'as required' analgesia is unsatisfactory as a response to pain relief for people with a learning disability and dementia. Staff need to be aware of and skilled in using non-pharmacological interventions that can be effective in aiding pain relief.

9

The Experiences
and Needs of Peers

As they grow older, people with a learning disability are increasingly likely to encounter friends and peers with dementia. The higher prevalence rate means that people with a learning disability may well encounter higher rates of dementia amongst their peers than do people without a learning disability. Although training is given to staff and sometimes family and carers about dementia in people with a learning disability, this is rarely the case for people with a learning disability themselves. Other residents or tenants may spend most of their days with the person with dementia. This will have an impact on their own lives and yet they may not have been given basic knowledge and skills to help them cope. It can be very frightening to see someone you know behaving in new and strange ways. It is important that people understand the reasons for the new behaviour.

People may also feel resentful that staff are spending more time with the person with dementia. I worked with a group of people who were living with people with dementia. Although they expressed care and concern for the people with dementia, they also expressed irritation that they were losing out on staff time. They agreed the person needed extra time but not at their expense.

There is evidence to suggest that improved understanding of the causes of changes in behaviour and needs associated with dementia amongst peers makes it less likely that the person with dementia will have to move (Antonangeli 1995). There are probably a number of reasons for this. Group pressure can be a powerful determinant of the way in which behaviours are tolerated. If members of the group are frightened by someone's behaviour or think that they should help themselves (when in fact they cannot), they may go on to reject and scapegoat them. It is also the case that the other tenants or residents may not understand the impact that their own behaviour has on the person with dementia. They might not appreciate that their responses may exacerbate situations and so encourage challenging behaviours in the person with dementia.

Wilkinson *et al.* (2004) found that when people who lived with the person with dementia were given training and information about the impact of dementia they were better able to tolerate the person's behaviour. One resident, for example, commented of another resident, 'He couldn't help it, it's an illness' (in reference to the night-time disturbance of a man with dementia: Wilkinson *et al.* 2004, p. 19). People are also able, if given the right information, to offer solutions (Kerr, Rae and Wilkinson 2002, p. 29) found evidence that the provision of targeted training and information enabled people to reflect on ways they could help and support the person with dementia:

- 'Calm them down a bit.'
- 'Do painting. Woodwork is most noisy workshop of all.'
- 'I wouldn't talk so loud around them – peaceful.'
- 'Be a bit calmer. More relaxed. Patient.'

There are some useful information booklets available which address the issue of dementia for people with a learning disability (Dodd, Turk and Christmas 2005; Kerr and Innes 2000).

I have used one of these booklets (*What is Dementia? A Booklet for Adults with a Learning Disability*: Kerr and Innes 2000) to provide information and opportunity for discussion with people who live with people with dementia. The following approach has proved successful:

- Preferably have no more then six people in the group.
- Have two members of staff so that communication issues are better dealt with.
- Photocopy each page of the booklet *What is Dementia?*. Make this into A3 size laminated posters and attach each photocopied page to a page of a flip chart. This provides a large central focus.

- Give each member of the group a copy of the booklet as well.

- It may be that people know the term 'Alzheimer's disease' already. This needs to be checked, as it will facilitate the conversation if you use a more familiar term. If dementia is a new term, it needs more emphasis.

- Spend about 20 minutes going through the first half of the booklet. After a break complete the booklet.

It is evident when carrying out training with groups of residents, tenants or day service users that there is a wealth of experience of the changes that occur when someone develops dementia.

- 'Their memory goes, they forget things.'

- 'When you talk to him he is completely confused. Imagines things happening but they are not.'

- 'He gets very confused, can't remember, get upset. In a wheelchair … used to walk, dancing, riding. Can't understand what he is saying. He talks faster … he gets mixed up … can't get perspective together.'

- 'Confused day and night.'

(Kerr *et al.* 2002 p. 29)

People need to be given an opportunity to express their anxieties and worries about the person with dementia. They also need strategies to help themselves and the person with dementia to cope.

Training sessions have also revealed a level of anxiety amongst people about their own likelihood of developing dementia. If they see so many older people developing the condition there is an understandable belief that the onset of the condition is an inevitable part of growing older.

Case Study 16

Michael, a man in his late thirties with Down's syndrome living in a village community with an ageing population, expressed this worry when he stated: 'Kate had Down's syndrome and she got dementia. Robert had Down's syndrome and he got dementia. Margaret has Down's syndrome and she has dementia. I have Down's syndrome'.

It is important to address the worries and anxieties of other people. Do not assume that just because people are not asking you the question they are not asking it of themselves. It is evident (Wilkinson *et al.* 2004) that a fairly small intervention can make a significant difference not only to the experiences and knowledge of people who live with those with dementia but also to the people with dementia themselves.

The provision of information and training is not without dilemmas. Someone with a learning disability living with someone with dementia may not be told of the diagnosis. There may be a number of reasons for this. Issues about confidentiality make decisions about whom to tell, and when, problematic. If the person with dementia does not know they have the condition and so will not have given consent for others to be told, staff need to be very careful about if, how and what information is given to others. Staff and carers may also not give information as a way of protecting the person without dementia from the experience of loss and anxiety. Staff and carers may also be struggling with their own grief and so do not feel able to cope with that of others. Another substantial reason, however, is often that staff and carers do not know where or how to begin with the explanation. The use of the booklets and training format given above may help staff to overcome this obstacle.

Dementia is a terminal condition. This means that people are going to see their friends die or move away to die. People will generally be older and may have known each other for much of their life. Many people will have known each other in a long-stay hospital or have lived together in supported housing for many years. People will need support and explanations about what is happening. It is of concern that often when people in the later stages are moved to hospital or a nursing facility their peers are not enabled to visit. Sometimes they are not even told where the person has gone. Comments such as:

- 'Bruce went away'. 'Where?' 'Don't know.'
- 'Don't know how she is now.'
- 'No one seen her since she went away.'

are indicative of a lack of continued involvement (Wilkinson, Kerr and Rae 2003, p. 28).

Often on further enquiry it is apparent that someone has visited, perhaps the person's best friend, but the information about the person who has moved has not been systematically related to people who know them. There is a danger that such lack of information means that the people who are left develop a fear of being sent away to some unknown and unwanted place where they will lose touch with friends and relatives.

Summary

Because of the higher prevalence rate of dementia amongst people with a learning disability, they are increasingly likely to live, work and socialise with people who have dementia. It is important, therefore, that they are given information that enables them to understand what is happening to their friend, other tenant or resident. This will help them to understand and cope with the changes that will inevitably occur. It might also help them to change some of their interactions so that they do not exacerbate the impact of the condition on the person with dementia. They may also develop strategies that help the person. Understanding the needs of the person with dementia may help them to come to terms with the fact that they will, sometimes, not receive the level of attention they had previously experienced.

The acknowledgement of the fact that someone has dementia does raise issues of confidentiality and disclosure that need to be addressed. It is also important that people are given an opportunity to express their own fears about their own vulnerability to the condition.

When people with dementia move to another setting, contact and the flow of information must be maintained. Lack of clear communication may lead to anxieties and misconceptions about what happens when people with dementia leave their home.

Supporting People to Eat Well

The onset of dementia will make eating and drinking increasingly difficult. Many people with a learning disability will already have experienced
problems with eating prior to the onset of dementia and strategies will
have been developed to minimise this. It is important that staff and carers
recognise that the onset of the condition means that many of these strategies will no longer be suitable and they need to develop new techniques
and responses.

It used to be thought that the weight loss that is often seen in people
with dementia was a direct result of the condition. This is not so. Although
in the latter stages of the condition people will inevitably lose weight, in
the early and mid stages this weight loss is clearly related to inadequate
support with eating and drinking. A study carried out by Watson (1994)
found that 50 per cent of people with dementia were malnourished.

Malnutrition and dehydration are very serious conditions. Poor nutrition and hydration may reduce the person's ability to cope, increase their
pain, generally diminish the quality of their life and ultimately may result
in death.

The following list is an indication of some of the more common and
profound consequences of under-nutrition and dehydration:

- apathy
- memory loss
- poor wound healing
- breathing difficulties
- skin problems and sores
- cardiac difficulties

- increased risk of infection
- prolonged complications after operation
- confusion
- musculoskeletal difficulties including weakness and poor coordination
- increased illness, disease and mortality.

The causes of malnutrition and dehydration amongst people with dementia are located in the changes that come about because of the condition and also because of inappropriate or even damaging events and practices in the physical, social and emotional environment. These all need to be addressed if the person is going to be supported well. These issues will be addressed under the following headings:

- how dementia affects the ability to eat and drink well
- using suitable food and routines
- developing suitable social, emotional and physical environments to aid eating and drinking.

How dementia affects the ability to eat and drink well

The following list of possible changes is no substitute for speech and language therapy involvement but it is provided as an essential backdrop to the advice that a speech and language therapist will give.

Practical or physical changes mean the person may:

- be unable to use cutlery
- have problems with tremor and be unable to get food to their mouth
- be unable to unwrap or peel food and may try to eat it wrapped
- be unable to sit for meals
- be extremely slow in eating.

Physiological changes mean the person may:

- have difficulty chewing
- have difficulty swallowing

- lose their sense of smell and taste
- lose their appetite
- have problems/pain with their teeth, gums and dentures
- show a preference for sweet food
- store food in their mouth.

Emotional and cognitive factors mean the person may:

- be easily distracted
- forget to eat or that they have eaten
- eat with their hands
- be unable to communicate hunger or thirst
- be unable to see and remember food or drink which is not directly in front of them
- eat non-food
- have difficulty making choices.

(Adapted from Hall (1994), reproduced in VOICES (1998, p. 17))

People with dementia are at significant risk of developing dysphagia. This is the term used to describe difficulties with eating, drinking and/or swallowing. These difficulties mean that the person is at great risk from choking on or inhaling their food and drink. It is essential, therefore, that expert, professional advice is sought. This will involve a referral to the speech and language therapist. Table 10.1 can be used to determine when a referral needs to be made. Ideally, however, the referral should be made when the diagnosis of dementia is given and should not wait until difficulties arise.

There will be other changes associated with ageing that may also impede the person's ability to eat and drink adequately. There is often a circular set of events that ensues. Conditions of ageing and/or learning disability lead to poor food or fluid intake. This then leads to the onset of conditions that further exacerbate the situation and further reduce the likelihood of the person eating and drinking enough.

Table 10.1 Dysphagia checklist

Please indicate if, and how often, the person exhibits the following:

(please photocopy this chart for continuous use)

	Never	*Sometimes*	*Always*
Coughing or choking during or after meal or drink times			
Dehydration			
Chest infections			
Urinary tract infections			
Change in voice quality – 'gurgly' or wet voice when speaking			
Drooling of saliva/food/fluid			
Nasal regurgitation			
Gasping for breath at meals			
Pockets of food around inside of mouth			
Fatigue at meal times – taking a long time to eat and drink			
More sleepy than usual after meal			
Suspected discomfort when swallowing			
Change of colour in the face			
Sounds of respiratory difficulty			
Rapid heart rate			
High temperature			

COMPLETED BY:
DATE:
NEXT COMPLETION DATE:

If you have responded in either the 'sometimes' or the 'always' column for any factor please contact your speech and language therapist to arrange a full assessment.

Source: Surrey and Borders NHS Partnership Trust (2006)

Dental problems

Problems with teeth and gums will increase with age. People with a learning disability are much more susceptible to dental decay and gum disease than the general population (Cumella *et al.* 2000). The impact of poor or inconsistent dental care earlier in life has a major impact in older age (Naidu *et al.* 2001). Many people with a learning disability have not been able to take adequate care of their teeth. Many had experiences of the dentist that have made them reluctant to seek further help. The consequence of this is often the presence of dental pain that inevitably affects the ability to eat.

Ear and hearing problems

Problems with hearing and ear pain will also have an impact on people's ability to concentrate on eating. People with a learning disability are twice as likely to have impacted ear wax than the general population (Fransman 2005). This can cause pain, discomfort, dizziness, noises in the ear and hearing loss. It can also lead to ear infection and, therefore, additional pain. A study carried out by Fransman (2005) found a correlation between the development of ear wax and the reduced ability to chew amongst people who did not have their back (molar) teeth. People with dementia also have problems with chewing. It may be that this also increases their susceptibility to impacted ear wax and consequent pain and hearing loss.

Urinary tract infections

Older people with a learning disability can experience higher levels of recurrent urinary tract infection than the general population (Janicki and Dalton 1998). The higher incidence of diabetes in people with a learning disability (Janicki and Dalton 1998), coupled with the reduced food and fluid intake as a consequence of dementia, also leaves the person at risk of a urinary infection (Holland and Benton 2004). The discomfort caused by urinary tract infection can be significant. This may well impede ability to sit and eat.

Constipation

The general slowing down of the gastrointestinal system in older age can lead to constipation as well as diarrhoea and irritable bowel syndrome. The pain associated with constipation can be severe and lead to many behaviours which can easily be misinterpreted and therefore mistreated (Lennox and Eastgate 2004). Of course, the susceptibility to become constipated is exacerbated by the fact that people with dementia, unless monitored and supported, may not be drinking sufficient water. They may also be less mobile. These two factors alone should alert staff to the possibility of someone with dementia becoming constipated.

Short-term memory problems

The onset of short-term memory problems has a profound effect on people's ability to remember whether they have eaten and drunk or not. It is not uncommon to see staff hand someone with dementia a cup of tea. The person will take the tea, place it on the table beside them and if it is out of sight for them it no longer exists. The tea will go cold and it is often the case that staff will come and take the cold tea away with comments such as 'Are you not thirsty?' Similarly food, particularly in hospital, may be placed on the table over the bed, with a cover on it. The person with dementia does not know what is under the cover and even if they can see the food, they may well not be able physically to eat the food. Staff will then take the cold food away.

It is also true that, for some people with dementia, there is an opposite experience, which is that far from forgetting or not being able to eat they will forget that they have eaten and constantly demand more food. This phenomenon may be the consequence of a number of factors. They may not be getting the message from their stomach to their brain that they are full. They may also see someone else eating and this acts as a trigger for their own desire to eat. The sound of staff clearing up the china and cutlery in the kitchen can serve as a reminder of food. The person hears the noise as an indication that food is being prepared and will appear back in the kitchen minutes after finishing their meal looking to eat again.

Using suitable food and routines

People's ability to eat different foods changes as the condition progresses. They will, increasingly, return to the ways of eating that they have known longest. When we learn to eat we move through sucking, eating with our fingers, eating with a spoon, then with a knife and fork. People with dementia will regress through these stages. Sometimes the regression will occur throughout the course of a day with the person being more able in the morning than at night. Increasingly this pattern will occur on a longer-term basis and the person will need to have finger foods and puréed foods provided at all meals. Offering meat and two vegetables may no longer be an option.

The use of finger foods helps to maintain independence in eating. It is important that the right food is given. The food should be easy to hold and also easy to swallow. Breaded chicken, for example, will not be easy to swallow and white bread will often become sticky and hard to manipulate.

Table 10.2 provides a useful list of possible finger foods that could be offered. Knowing the likes and dislikes of each individual should result in priority being given to some of these, and others, being added.

People will need their food made progressively easier to swallow. There should be an increasing use of soft but textured food such as breakfast cereals soaked in warm milk to soften the texture and fruit and vegetables that are well cooked with no stones or skins, and dairy products such as yoghurt and cheese dishes with sauces. Eventually the person may have to move on to puréed food. It is recognised, however, that 'it is difficult to achieve a nutritionally adequate diet from puréed food unless great care is taken to monitor the food eaten and to plan a varied diet' (VOICES 1998, p. 38).

The following should be taken into consideration when using puréed food:

- Be careful when blending food that the texture is smooth.
- Be careful not to over-dilute the food as this will reduce the nutritional value.
- Be aware that if the food is too modified it may not be recognisable to the person.

Table 10.2 Finger foods

Bread and cereals

Buttered toast fingers	Gingerbread
Buttered muffins	Cereal bars
Buttered buns	Won-tons
Tea bread	Sandwiches
Drop scones	Crackers and butter
Small pittas	Fruit loaf
Rolls and butter	Waffles
Buttered crumpet fingers	Chapatis
French toast	Prawn crackers

Meat, fish, cheese and other protein alternatives

Sliced meat, cut up into pieces	Chicken pieces from moist breast
Sausages and frankfurters	Hamburgers
Slices of pork pie	Quiche
Fish fingers and fishcakes	Fish sticks or crab sticks
Smoked mackerel slices	Vegetable or soya sausages
Vegetable burgers or fingers	Quartered boiled egg
Cheese on toast	Cheese cubes
Fried bean curd cubes	Pizza

Vegetables

Carrot sticks or coins, cooked	Broccoli spears, cooked
Brussels sprouts, cooked	Green beans, cooked
Chips	Potato waffles
New potatoes	Sweet potato coins
Fried battered onion rings	Fried plantain
Fried, crumbled whole mushrooms	Sliced cucumber
Quartered tomato	Celery sticks

Fruit

Banana	Grapes
Strawberries	Sliced apple or pear
Melon	Mandarin orange segments

Snacks

Dried apricots or prunes (stones removed)	Muesli bars
Jelly cubes	Marmite on toast
Ice cream in cones	Pate on toast
Peanut butter sandwiches	Savoury snacks

Source: Adapted from Ford (1996), reproduced in VOICES (1998)

- Make sure that puréed food is still energy dense by adding calorie-rich foods such as butter and cream.
- Purée each part of the meal separately: this way different colours and flavours will remain.
- Sometimes it is helpful to rearrange the food to look like its original form, for example puréed carrot could be moulded into a carrot shape.
- Puréed vegetables can be thickened with a sauce for some people.

The changing needs of people's diet mean that staff will often have to be proactive in determining what people eat. It may also be that staff have to actively intervene in the choices being made by the person.

It is not uncommon to see people at their day service queuing up with everyone else and having food put on their plate that they can neither recognise, manipulate nor enjoy. Staff must be aware that this may well mean that they are not eating enough. Actively recording what is eaten using the chart provided in Table 10.3 will help to reduce this risk and develop a proactive approach to meal times. Everyone involved in supporting people to eat and drink well should keep the chart shown in Table 10.3, which is taken from *Down's Syndrome and Dementia: Workbook for Staff* (Dodd *et al.* 2006, p. 87).

Table 10.3 Food and fluid intake chart

Day/date time	What food was offered?	What food was eaten?	What drink was offered?	What drink was drunk?

Source: Dodd, Kerr and Fern (2006)

What is important is that the person eats and drinks enough. To an extent the quantity, whilst not overriding the quality, needs to become more of a focus for staff. This may mean that it is acceptable to eat foods that previously would have been discouraged. People with dementia, for example, seem to have a preference for sweet foods. These might have previously been discouraged but this stricture should, provided there are no medical contra-indications, be slackened. The liking for sweet things means that often people will prefer to eat their pudding rather than the savoury main course. Foods that have been a favourite may no longer be so. They may show a liking for foods that they used to like many years ago before the onset of the dementia. A preference for spicy foods that have more distinctive taste may also be apparent. These changes in taste are the result of the changes that are occurring in the brain.

There is a change not only in taste but also in the amount and frequency of eating. People may want to eat smaller meals or snack continuously. There is no point in continuing to demand that the person continues with their previous diet and routines if there is as a consequence reduced nutrition and challenging behaviour. Someone who becomes increasingly sedentary or restless will have different energy requirements at different times of the day. So a big breakfast followed by a main meal at lunchtime and a light snack for supper or tea may be appropriate for the sedentary person but the person who paces may need to eat fairly constantly. The pattern of three set meals a day will often have to be abandoned in favour of a more person-centred approach to providing food and opportunities to eat.

Adaptations need to be made. This can be difficult for peers to witness. To see someone being allowed to eat or offered foods that were previously discouraged because they were fattening or not healthy enough, and seeing staff cooking special meals or seeing someone being allowed to eat anywhere but at the table can cause discontent. This is a reason for working with friends, peers and other residents or tenants, perhaps using the booklets referred to in Chapter 9, to help them understand the reasons behind these changes.

For staff and carers the challenge is to find ways of helping the person to consume food in a way that still retains their dignity and respects their choices as far as is reasonably possible.

Case study 17

Molly is a 54-year-old woman with Down's syndrome and a diagnosis of dementia. She lived in supported accommodation with three other people. Molly was extremely agitated and paced up and down all day. Attempts to get her to sit down were fairly unsuccessful. At meal times she would sit briefly, maybe eat one mouthful and then would set off to walk about. The consequence of this behaviour meant that she was losing weight rapidly. Not only was she burning off fat by her constant activity but also she was not replacing this by eating enough. She was also developing skin problems and was increasingly confused.

Staff had tried a number of strategies, all of which had failed. Discussions about when and where to move Molly to a nursing environment were being set up. Molly's key worker was concerned that such a move would not be in Molly's best interest. She tried a new approach. She made Molly an apron with two large pockets. She also made a number of large pouches, in bright orange waterproof material. These pouches were placed in the pockets, filled with food that Molly liked (not necessarily the healthy food previously encouraged).

As Molly walked about she ate the food that she could see sticking out of the top of the pouches. As the pouches became empty staff would refill them. Molly regained her previous weight before any decisions were made about hospitalisation or a move to a nursing home. Molly continued to live in her supported house.

This case study underlines the need to try new things and not to try to force the person to keep to inappropriate routines. The important thing is to work out when the person is most lucid and most able to eat and drink and to make sure that it is at this time that they are offered their most nutritious meal. It demonstrates how necessary it is to make sure that the person is regularly weighed. If there is weight loss the dietician must be consulted.

The need to monitor people's food and fluid intake becomes increasingly important. Adults need to drink at least one and a half litres of fluid a day and to have a balanced diet throughout the course of the day and night. Do not assume that just because there is an empty cup or plate that the person has drunk or eaten the contents. Everyone involved in the person's fluid and food intake should record what has been consumed and also make sure that a named person monitors this information. The danger, otherwise, is that assumptions are made that someone has eaten at their day centre because they are not eating at night or that they are not hungry at lunchtime because they had a big breakfast. If this is not recorded and the person cannot remember, then there is a strong possibility that they will not be eating or drinking enough.

Developing suitable social, emotional and physical environments to aid eating and drinking

Meal times are not just a source of gaining food and drink. They are also important social events. They often have emotional and social significance. Babies learn early on that food is associated with their mother and so with company. Throughout our lives this association continues. Meal times provide an opportunity to relate to someone else. When someone develops dementia they become more needy of the presence of significant others and this is particularly necessary at meal times. It is important, therefore, that a member of staff or carer sits with the person during meal times.

Malone (1996) comments that 'Increased social activity results in increased eating behaviour and it may be that the social environment is as important as the actual food being eaten. Thus any environmental manipulation, whether physical or social, which stimulates socialisation, is desirable'.

The presence of someone who can prompt the person to eat aids the process. Telling the person what is on the plate and where it is will be helpful and reduce anxiety. If the person has problems getting food into their mouth, gently assisting them to lift and direct the spoon or touching their mouth can help. It is important that the staff member is not distracted and disturbed during this time. A good way to reduce distractions and help concentration to aid eating is for staff to eat with the person. This helps give the person cues and they can mirror the staff behaviour. It also feels more normal to share a meal than to be watched whilst you eat.

This can be very time consuming. Someone with dementia will often take about 35–40 minutes to eat their meal, and this means that a staff member needs to be free for that length of time. It is often the case that the food will need to be reheated. This will not only make the food more palatable but also bring back the smell of the food, which will help to stimulate the person's appetite.

It is disturbing to discover that there are some authorities that provide food described as 'cook and chill'. This food is cooked centrally and then distributed and reheated by the staff. This food cannot be reheated once it has gone cold. It is cold within 20 minutes. The person with dementia is then presented with a cold, congealed meal that is offensive and often inedible. This means that the person either is going to have to eat something that others would reject or will simply go without. This policy is not suitable for people with dementia.

Here are some other environmental considerations that will aid eating:

- Have a calm environment free from distractions.

- Keep the noise levels down. Many places, not just day services but even people's own homes, are much too noisy at meal times.

- Use good lighting over the meal table so that the person can see well what is on their plate.

- Use plain plates. People with dementia have problems seeing things in three dimensions. They will see changes in colour as changes in level. Patterns on the plate will look as if they are standing proud. People may well mistake the pattern for food and will try to pick it up.

- For similar reasons use plain tablecloths or mats. These should be in a contrasting colour to the plates so that it easier to distinguish the plates. Having plates with a dark line round the edge can also help recognition.

- Finding the right music to play at meal times can sometimes aid eating. A study carried out in Sweden found that people with dementia in nursing homes were 'less irritable, anxious and depressed and ate more when music was played at meal times' (Ragnoskog 1994). The wrong music, of course, will increase agitation and impede eating well. Some people (Goldsmith 1996) would argue that any music is adding clutter to the environment and is potentially distracting so should be avoided. The best advice is to try it and see. Staff should know the music that the person finds most relaxing.

- Use supportive chairs. Because people with a learning disability live in ordinary housing, as far as possible, they will also have ordinary seating, unless contra-indicated by their needs. When someone develops dementia they will, as stated earlier, have problems with swallowing. They will also often sit at an angle, leaning to one side. Clearly if someone is not sitting straight then swallowing becomes more difficult; there is an increased risk of liquid and food going into the lungs and therefore an increased risk of the person developing aspirant pneumonia. Seats that support the person to sit straight and support their head are essential. If it is not possible to buy a purpose-built chair then at least improvise with cushions.

- The social, emotional and physical environment at night may be more conducive to supporting people to eat well. The environment is more likely to be calm and noise free and the person may get one-to-one attention at 4 o'clock in the morning rather than 4 o'clock in the afternoon. This is not to suggest that people are deliberately woken to eat but, as people with dementia tend to have disturbed nights, this might be a more positive response than trying to get them back to bed.

In the later stages of the condition people will find it increasingly difficult to eat and drink. They will lose weight and often will appear not to be interested in food. This does not mean that they do not need to eat or drink. Certainly I have heard of people in the late stage of the condition being left with no food or drink. When questioned, staff have said that people with dementia in late stage are beyond eating and drinking. This must be challenged. There are a number of reasons for the increase in problems:

- Chewing becomes more difficult.

- Fluid control and swallowing become problematic and a major safety issue for the person.

- Memory loss means that the person loses the ability to recognise food.

- They no longer understand the need to eat, not recognising the signals that tell them they are hungry or thirsty.
- They can completely forget the way to eat.
- The person may experience a return of reflex actions (e.g. sucking, biting) that interfere with eating.
- The person may appear to resist attempts to help them eat but this may be because of the problems listed above. It does not mean that they should not be offered food.

Specialist advice and help should have been sought earlier on in the progression of the condition. It is now absolutely essential that the speech and language therapist, the occupational therapist and the dietician be involved.

Below is some advice; it is, however, no substitute for getting an assessment done by the appropriate professionals.

- Although drinking is essential, it is also associated with risk of chest infections, choking or asphyxiation. Anxiety about the possibility of choking can lead to a reduction in the amount of fluids offered. It is important, however, to give plenty of fluids and to supervise the person to make sure that they actually drink safely. They may require thickened fluids or modifications in the way they are given fluids, for example using a shallow cup or teaspoon.
- Instructing the person to 'chew' or 'swallow' and touching the central bud of the top lip with the spoon can stimulate swallowing.
- An upright position is needed for feeding and drinking. The head of the bed should be elevated to the highest tolerable position or the person should remain in their chair. The person should sit upright for approximately 30 minutes after eating to reduce the risk of inhaling following reflux (indigestion or release of swallowed air mixed with stomach juices). Minimise the amount of movement during that time, so toileting or moving chairs should not occur if possible.
- The mouth should be checked and cleaned of any remaining food after eating as the person may forget or have had problems swallowing.

- There is a huge range of aids and adaptations available to help with eating, drinking and reducing mess. These include special beakers, adapted cutlery, plate guards and non-slip mats, blenders and protective covers for clothing.

- If feeding becomes very difficult, it may become necessary to consider feeding the person intravenously or by the use of percutaneous endoscopic gastrosomy (PEG feeding).

The decision to use PEG is not straightforward and should be made only after multidisciplinary discussions with all interested parties.

There are no simple answers or single solutions. It is imperative that a thorough assessment is carried out before any decisions are made. The decisions must include not only the preferences and quality of life for the person with dementia but also the type of support available to staff in relation to training and advice.

Guidelines for helping people to eat well

The following guidelines might be a useful sheet to have displayed for carers and staff, to remind them of the very basic requirements if someone with learning disability and dementia is going to be supported to eat and drink.

- Staff should be present and involved at meal times.

- Make sure the environment is calm.

- Review times of meals to ensure they are appropriately spaced.

- To avoid disorientation, tables should not be set more than 30 minutes before a meal.

- Put only one course on the table at a time. Do not use service trays.

- Finger food should be served when necessary.

- People should be allowed to chose where they sit.

- When serving soup, offer a choice of cup or bowl, if this is possible.

- The same carer should be with the person throughout the meal.

- Make sure the person has clean glasses, clean dentures and hearing aid.

- Make sure the person is in an upright position.
- The carer should sit at eye level or slightly below and either immediately in front or slightly to one side.
- Small mouthfuls – but enough for the person to feel food in their mouth.
- Assist but never force.
- Give adequate time for swallowing.
- Do not talk to anyone else.
- Give verbal prompts; talk clearly, gently and firmly.
- Discourage the person from talking with their mouth full.

Summary

People with dementia have increasing difficulty with eating and drinking. It is essential that those who support them get advice from relevant professionals, speech and language therapists, dieticians and occupational therapists.

Attention must be given to the social, emotional and physical environment in which people eat. The environment should be calm and distraction free. The amount, type and consistency of food offered must be monitored and adjusted to the changing abilities of the person as the condition progresses. The use of finger foods and blended foods should be introduced as appropriate. It is also important that people are given time and attention at meal times. It may also be necessary to move from present routines and be prepared to provide food at different times of the day. Providing a way in which the person can carry food with them may be a simple but effective solution to some people's reluctance to sit and eat. There is a myriad of ways in which people can be supported to eat well. Staff should try these before decisions are made about the use of PEG feeding. Decisions to use this intervention must be based on assessment of the person's needs, history and personality, and the levels of staff training and availability.

11

Creating Supportive
Physical Environments

We are all supported, controlled, enabled and disabled by the various physical environments that we use for work, pleasure and accommodation. The same is true for people with dementia, although to a considerable extent they are even more influenced by the environment in which they find themselves. People without dementia usually have the ability to manipulate their environment so that it can serve rather than impede. This is not so true for people with dementia; it is even less true if they have a learning disability as well as dementia. When working with people with a learning disability and dementia, the potentially disabling effect of the environment must be taken into account and rectified.

This chapter will describe ways in which design and adaptations to the environment can compensate, enable or at the very least avoid the imposition of further disabling experiences induced by the environment. It is important to remember that people who have dementia will be older. People with Down's syndrome who develop dementia often in their middle age will also be affected by the conditions of older age. When considering the design and features of the environment, therefore, it is necessary to consider the impact of ageing as well dementia.

There is now a substantial body of literature on the requirements of an environment suitable for people with dementia (Brawley 1997; Calkins 1988; Cantley and Wilson 2003; Cohen and Day 1993; Cohen and Weisman 1991; Judd, Marshall and Phippen 1998; Utton 2007). This body of work has informed the ideas and recommendations given in this chapter.

A useful way to think about the type of design and features that are essential to an environment for people with a learning disability and dementia is to use the following criteria. The environment must be:

- calm and stress-free
- predictable and make sense
- familiar
- suitably stimulating
- safe.

Calm and stress-free

The environment can very easily become stressful for people with dementia. Stress caused by noise levels is common. People with dementia have difficulty with even ordinary levels of noise in their environment. As we age, our hearing becomes impaired. A condition that results in the impairment of selective frequency hearing, presbycusis, reduces our ability to discriminate between different sounds such as conversation and background noise. Additionally people with dementia, because of their cognitive impairment and consequent short-term memory loss, often cannot decide which noise is relevant. All noise goes into our ears but we then decide what to attend to. If people with dementia cannot make that decision, they do not know which noises to cut out. This can be extremely disturbing and distressing. Buildings need to be designed to reduce noise levels. High-pitched roofs, large open-plan areas, uncarpeted, hard surfaced flooring can all amplify rather than reduce noise.

Staff need also to be aware of the many things that contribute to the level of noise in the environment. Televisions and radios, often being listened to by other residents, tenants or staff, should be turned off unless absolutely necessary. If they need to be on, then the volume should be turned as low as is acceptable. The noise of washing machines, vacuum cleaners, dishwashers and other electrical appliances may seem innocuous to the person without dementia but may be overwhelming for the person with dementia. Hiatt (1995) has suggested that noise for people with dementia is the equivalent of stairs for people using wheelchairs. It is an illuminating exercise to simply stand in an environment and count how many different noises there are. People without dementia will often be unaware of the extent of the noise 'clutter'.

The use of the right music can reduce agitation. Music should not be played all day (it will agitate the staff as well as the person with dementia if it is constantly played). As indicated in Chapter 6 on therapeutic interventions, the optimum time to have music playing is 20 minutes in one hour.

A calm environment should not be too busy. Design should enable one activity to be taking place without the disturbance from others. Often activities in day services take place in large rooms where there are a number of people, many engaged in different activities. Apart from the obvious noise implications this also adds movement and stimuli to the environment. The need to reduce the stimuli in the environment also requires staff and others to slow down. People rushing about will agitate the person with dementia. Many buildings are designed in a way that requires staff to be monitoring more than one area at a time and this may lead them to rush from one room to another.

The provision of care and support should ideally be within a setting where there are no more than eight people resident. Above this number the dynamic becomes too much and the person is at risk of being agitated and further confused. The issue of increased numbers of people in the environment is particularly relevant and problematic at meal times when, particularly in day services, large numbers of people often come together to eat. Every effort should be made to have a design that enables meals to be taken in quiet, homely environments that are calm.

Predictable and make sense

The memory impairment characteristic of dementia combines with visual losses to make the environment often unpredictable and as a consequence it often does not make sense. One of the functions lost is the ability to see things in three dimensions. This means that people with dementia will erroneously believe that changes in colour are also changes in level. It is common to see people with dementia trying to step over things that are actually not raised. They will try to step over the metal strip between rooms and over patterns on the carpet and vinyl flooring. A dark square on light flooring may look like a hole that a person needs to walk round or avoid. The flooring not only does not make sense, thus causing increased agitation and distress, but also increases the possibility that people will fall.

Small patterns may suggest that there are objects on the floor. People will often bend to try to pick these up. This, again, is likely to cause agitation as it does not make sense and it will increase the likelihood of the person toppling over.

Case study 18

Caroline, a woman in her late sixties with dementia, lived in supported accommodation. She loved having baths with bubbles, music and candles. As her dementia progressed, bathing became one of her favourite activities.

One day, however, Caroline refused to get into the bath. The staff discussed this development and discovered that this happened when one member of staff was bathing her but not when another was. The first reaction to this was to assume that the differences in her behaviour were related to the practices of the people helping her with her bathing.

Further enquiry revealed that the member of staff who was having difficulties placed the bath mat on the floor before Caroline got into the bath. The second staff member placed the mat on the floor after Caroline was in the bath and just before she got out. What was clearly causing the problem was the mat. It looked to Caroline like a big hole in front of the bath. There was nothing that would induce her to step into the void. When she got out of the bath the second staff member had the towel round her and she did not see the edges of the mat.

Problems with three-dimensional vision can also impact on other aspects of the environment. Patterned wallpaper can look as though things are in relief, so people may be tempted to try to pick things off the wall. Similarly tablecloths and crockery may appear to have things on them in relief. The person with dementia may try to pick the patterns off plates. This obviously can be distressing and also interferes with their eating.

A critical issue for people with dementia is stairs. Problems with three-dimensional vision make negotiating stairs highly problematic. Buildings for people with dementia should be single storey. The use of lifts is not an answer. People will be disturbed by the enclosure, by the changes in flooring and cannot usually use them by themselves.

Bathroom floors do generally pose a problem for people with dementia. A shiny floor might look like a pool of water. The flooring that is in most bathrooms in supported housing, residential and nursing homes tends to be 'non-slip' flooring that not only is shiny but also has shiny flecks in it. The result is a highly shiny and watery-looking surface. It is common to see people with dementia refusing to go into the bathroom for this reason. The flooring should be matt and preferably the same colour as the carpet in the room that leads into it. This then avoids the problems with changing colours.

The buffing up of vinyl flooring in day services and other settings where people with dementia want to walk around further exacerbates the problem of shiny floors. The sight of someone in their day service walking tentatively with their back pressed to the wall indicates their fear of the flooring, which they probably see as a pool of water. Of course the environment no longer makes sense and is as a consequence often very distressing.

Sight is the most important sense for acquiring information (Julian and Verriest 1997). With age, however, this important sense becomes impaired. Neural changes, which are associated with dementia and are present in older age, will lead to visual difficulties (Koncelik 2003). It is estimated that we require three times the level of illumination when we are older, compared to when we were in our twenties (Pollock 2007). Adaptation to changes in light is slowed in older age (Stuart-Hamilton 2000). It is essential, therefore, to provide adequate and appropriate lighting to enable people with dementia to see and orientate themselves in their environment.

Blurred vision occurs in the ageing eye and the eye gradually loses its ability to focus at close range. This generally begins at the age of 40 and focusing at close range is almost completely impossible by the age of 65 (Pollock 2007). This means that small objects or signs become difficult to see without reading glasses. Blurred vision also affects distant objects. This not only affects the ability to watch things like television, but also has an impact on mobility and balance.

As we age, the yellowing of the eyes means that we see the colours at the top end of the spectrum better than those at the bottom end. Red, orange and yellow are more easily seen than indigo and violet. This problem is exacerbated by the onset of dementia. It is helpful, therefore, to paint things that you want to be highly visible one of the colours at the top end of the spectrum. This should be combined with contrasting colours as this significantly aids differentiation and so makes features more obvious.

The painting of toilet doors red will not necessarily mean that the person with dementia recognises red as the colour of toilet doors. It will, however, mean that they will be better able to see the red door and consequently they will be more likely to be drawn towards it.

Within the toilet and bathing areas, the issue of contrast is very important. Often these settings are in pale and white colours to promote the concept of a hygienic area. Without use of contrast, the person will not be able to see the toilet easily. The floor, toilet, toilet seat and wall all need to contrast to ensure the person can easily identify and use the toilet. The use of a red toilet seat with the lid left up can help people to recognise where to sit. Although red would be the colour of choice, the use of other colours from the top end of the spectrum, used in contrast with the wall, may work equally well.

Memory problems mean that the person cannot remember where their room is, where the toilet is, where the kitchen is. This is a frightening experience. It is easy to imagine this situation by considering how you would react and cope in a hotel that did not have numbers on the doors. All the doors will look the same. This is true of most ordinary houses and institutional provision. The person without dementia can remember that their door is at the end of the landing or corridor. The person with dementia is just faced with an array of doors that all look the same. Often they will respond by entering the first door they come to. The consequent distress to themselves if they find themselves in a cupboard, or the wrong room, and if it is someone else's room the distress to that person, can lead to increased anxiety for everyone and 'challenging behaviour' by the person with dementia. Good signage is critical. People need to be shown what is behind a door. Have pictures of toilets on the toilet doors. The matchstick symbols in general use are not suitable: these mean nothing to someone whose memory has taken them back to a time before such images were used. The picture should be bold and easy to see. This means that it needs to be placed at a lower level than usual. As we age the eye muscles weaken. This affects the direct field of vision and reduces the ability of the eyeball to look directly ahead. The spine also shortens with age. These two factors, combined with the fact that many people with a learning disability, and particularly people with Down's syndrome, are below average height means that significant information and signage need to be placed at an appropriate height to provide information.

The use of signage to enable people either to recognise or simply to be drawn towards their bedroom is imperative. Placing on the door pictures that have significance can help. Another useful feature is to have a Perspex box on the door with a sliding front. Objects that will attract the person with dementia can be placed in the box.

Case study 19

An ingenious piece of signage was designed for a man who constantly went into another tenant's room. His room was further along the landing but he always entered the first door he came to. Staff who supported him knew that when he had lived at home he would accompany his father regularly to the local pub. The staff made an exact replica of the sign and hung it outside of his bedroom. This worked like magic. The man walked straight to the sign and then entered his room. He was not, as one might imagine, disappointed not to find the bar and his dad inside. He simply responded to something that was very familiar in his long-term memory and then was pleased and relaxed to be in his bedroom.

Placing pictures on kitchen cupboard doors to indicate what is in each cupboard is helpful. This needs a level of caution, however. I recommended this to the people who lived with a woman who had dementia. Some months later I was informed by one of the tenants that this did not work because the people without dementia took no notice of the pictures and put things randomly into cupboards. The use of Perspex or glass fronts on cupboard doors can circumvent this problem.

People with dementia are affected by the fading light in the afternoon. This phenomenon, known as 'sun downing', means that the person sees their environment differently. It becomes less predictable and does not make sense. They can become agitated and may well be particularly 'challenging' at this time. The use of light-sensitive time switches or even mechanised time switches, which are set to come on three to four hours before sunset, can help to counteract this effect. The use of daylight lighting with no glare is most effective. There should be dimmer switches that staff can then use when it is time for people to go to bed.

If possible there should be different rooms for different tasks. If a room is used for more than one task or activity, it is important to remove visual cues from previous activities and make sure that there are clear cues for the activity that is intended. Mirrors can present people with dementia with a confusing and frightening experience. Because of the loss of recent memory the person no longer sees themselves as the age they are. If they look into a mirror the person they see will not tally with their own self-image, which is of a younger person. This does not make sense. It is not hard to imagine how disturbing this can be. This is particularly the case at night when shadows are reflected in the mirrors on wardrobes and dressing tables.

Case study 20

Pamela is a 54-year-old woman with Down's syndrome and a diagnosis of dementia. The onset of the dementia had led to a change in her sleeping pattern. She began to wake at night. Initially she was not disturbed by this but just needed reassurance from the staff. Pamela then began to become very agitated when she woke. She would scream that people were in her room and they were dancing on the end of her bed. Staff would try to reassure her but as soon as they left the room she became distressed again about the 'intruders'. On investigation it transpired that Pamela had a dressing table at the end of her bed. This had three mirrors, a large central one with two hinged smaller mirrors on each side. It was clear that what Pamela could see was her own reflection in the mirrors. This appeared to her as a number of people dancing. The more agitated she became, shouting and waving them away, the more they 'danced'. The simple device of covering the mirror at night removed all agitation.

It is particularly disturbing to reflect on the possibility that Pamela's behaviour appeared to be hallucinatory, and antipsychotic or sedative medication might have been prescribed.

People shouting 'Get that man out of my room' or 'People are trying to kill me' can sound hallucinatory when in fact these reactions may well be misidentifications that require the removal or covering of a mirror. It is not always necessary or indeed desirable to remove mirrors. People may be able to recognise themselves during the day but not at night. The decisions about when to remove the mirror will need to be linked to the progression of the condition. I was told a cautionary tale about a woman who became very distressed by the person (herself reflected in the mirror) who she thought was sitting in her bedroom watching television with her. Staff removed the mirror. The next time the lady opened her bedroom door she screamed, 'Where is my room?' It transpired that the removal of the mirror, an important artefact in her life and well remembered, had made the room not look like hers.

Pictures with reflective glass can also cause reflections. Windows without curtains drawn when it is dark outside can also cause people to see their own reflection as an intruding stranger.

Familiar

Because of the 'roll-up' memory described in Chapter 4 on different realities, people will not recognise things that were not around at the age they are now experiencing. Someone who is 70 years old but whose reality is now the 1950s will have difficulty making sense of much modern equipment and many contemporary objects and features. The use of traditional-looking equipment can enhance the maintenance of skills and reduce agitation.

Taps are a good example of this. The use of mixer taps can be very confusing: coronation or cross-bar taps would be more familiar to someone with dementia.

For the person to be able to clean themselves after using the toilet, the use of traditional toilet-roll holders is also recommended. The newer toilet paper dispensers are not familiar to people who are relying on their long-term memory to make sense of things. If these things are not in place, the person may require carer interventions to assist them.

The use of traditional-style lamps, chairs, clocks and kitchen utensils should be encouraged. In residential settings, the development of a room that is furnished with things from the past can prove to be very relaxing because of its familiarity. It is, of course, important to know which stage in the past needs to be replicated.

It is disturbing to see institutional design for people with dementia, which does not look homely and familiar as a place to live. Long corridors and large communal spaces do not give a message that this place is where people live. It will give a message that this is probably a place of transition, an airport, a hotel, a hospital or a school. For many people with a learning disability it may well be that it looks and feels like the long-stay hospital where they lived in the past. This would be familiar but might not be welcome.

Suitably stimulating

The environment needs to provide a level of stimulation that does not leave the person distressingly alone and feeling ignored. As described elsewhere throughout this book the person with a learning disability and dementia can become quickly stressed by over-stimulation. The environment must therefore not be too noisy or have too much activity. The provision of small quiet areas is essential. These should provide opportunities for peaceful, calm activity. The use of large windows that give good ground-floor outside views can provide suitable stimulation. The provision of gardens, which encourages as well as enables people to go outside, will provide a level of suitable stimulation that is not only suitable but also healthy.

Safe

There are a number of safety issues that need to be taken into account within the environment. People with a learning disability and dementia will go out of doors, even if they have no clear purpose in doing so. A door is something we go though. The person without dementia can make an informed decision about when and why they might go through doors; the person with dementia will often simply respond to the trigger that the door gives and will go through. This can present safety risks.

It is important that the design of the building does not encourage people to exit through doors when it is not safe to do so. Disguising doors by painting them the same colour as the walls can be a way to remove the trigger. Running the handrail across the door so that there is a continuous line can help to reduce the visual impact of the door.

The doors that cause the most problems are fire doors. These are often deliberately placed in a conspicuous place, often at the end of a long corridor, where they allow light into the corridor through the glass panels. The fire door quite literally becomes the light at the end of the tunnel. The person with dementia will be drawn towards this and will then inevitably exit through to the outside that is visible and accessible.

The way to deal with this is to change the appearance of the fire door from a door into a window. Hang a dark cloth on the bottom half, with a section cut out to expose the push bar, and then hang curtains on the top half. This simple change can enable people who endlessly leave their day service through the fire door to continue to attend. It can prevent people being moved into locked accommodation and, as importantly, it can reduce stress levels for both staff and people with dementia.

It is important to involve the local fire department early on in decisions about fire doors. If the department is made aware of the rationale for changes, they may well agree to the doors being relocated and will be ready to accept the changes to the appearance of the fire door.

The use of locked doors and even restraint can become practices used to contain and restrict people who want to walk. Restraint is illegal except when particular legal measures have been taken; also keeping people behind locked doors with no opportunity for free access to the outside can be a source of anxiety and distress. The use of simple changes to the environment can make it safer for people to walk about and even reduce or stop the habit of going through certain doors.

A high prevalence of joint, postural or muscular problems that will affect mobility (McClean 2000) is found in older people with a learning disability, as in the general population. For people with Down's syndrome this will occur at an earlier age, perhaps even from their forties onwards. This is compounded by reduced sensation in the feet, which helps control balance. This affects the ability to adjust to changes in gradient or the depth of a walking surface. It is important therefore that floors are level. Often when there is an extension built or a wall is taken down, the difference in floor level requires a slight slope. This should be avoided.

Design should also enable people to walk about. There is something of an irony in attitudes to people walking about or wandering. Staff often have concerns about what activities to provide for people with dementia and yet one activity that many clearly enjoy is seen as a problem and one to be discouraged. Buildings need to be designed in such a way that they enable people to walk about. Walking about outside is particularly beneficial. This requires attention to be given to the development of suitable gardens.

Gardens for people with dementia

When thinking about the development of environments for people with dementia it is important to consider external as well as internal space. In Chapter 7 on challenging behaviour, the recognition that people with dementia need to walk about and not be labelled as 'wanderers' was developed. If people are going to be enabled to walk about, enjoy fresh air, get sun for the production of Vitamin D and generally experience a calm, stress-free and enjoyable activity, then the provision of a suitable garden becomes an imperative. With imagination a small area can be turned into a suitably stimulating garden for people with dementia.

The following guidelines, taken and adapted from *Designing Gardens for People with Dementia* by Annie Pollock (2001), are not comprehensive but should provide sufficient information for the development of a useful and pleasant outdoor space.

Boundary fences

- Do not make these too high. There is a temptation to make the fences high to keep people in but this will also make it appear like a prison. It might also encourage fit people to try to climb over to see what is on the other side. Fences of 1.6 metres are usually more than adequate.

- Design the fence to discourage climbing. Have vertical poles with the horizontal struts on the outside.

- Plant bushes along the fence to disguise it.

- If there has to be a gate to the outside, disguise it so that it looks like the fence.

Paths

- The gradient should be no more than 1:20.
- The path should lead round and through the garden and return to the beginning.
- Avoid abrupt changes of direction or dead ends. A figure of eight will provide variety and will always return the person to the beginning.
- The path should be wide enough for a wheelchair and allow others to pass.
- Think about providing a handrail if the gradient changes or simply to give people some reassurance every so often on as they walk around.
- It is a good idea to place a swing gate on the path. This gives people a sense of travel. This can be placed at the point where the path is bordered by shrubs. Another possibility is to place the gate within a pergola. A simple swing gate with hinges to allow it to open either way would be excellent.
- Make sure the path passes through different areas. Areas of lawn, areas of shrub bedding and patio areas will provide variety.
- Use raised kerbs where the path runs between planting beds to avoid soil spillage on to the path.

Resting places

- It is important that the garden does not become a 'parade ground' with people walking round and round.
- Provide resting places. These should be set sufficiently off the path to provide space for a solid bench and a wheelchair.
- Make sure these areas are sheltered from the wind, but place them so that they catch some sun.
- It may be worth having sheltered alcoves for people to be completely out of the wind and light rain.
- Make sure that the benches are placed with an interesting view. Provide bird tables, sculptures, interesting plants and a safe water feature.

Garden furniture and features

- Seating must be solid and comfortable. Make sure the arms have rounded ends for leaning on.

- Provide some good solid bird tables.

- Large stable pots and tubs will provide interest and colour and the possibility of all year round planting.

- Pergolas are a good way to divide one area from another.

- Use trellising to grow plants on and to provide shelter and privacy.

- In larger gardens consider the use of greenhouses, summerhouses and other objects of interest. I know of one garden that had an old car in it. This was a delight for some of the men who lived in the house.

- Rabbit hutches and aviaries should be considered.

- Provide raised potting tables and tubs so that people in wheelchairs can easily access them. These are also ideal for people who find bending difficult.

Plants and flowers

- Use plants that provide seasonal interest, colour and texture. Group colours together. Too much colour can be confusing.

- Choose plants that were popular 40 years ago.

- Use plants that encourage wildlife.

- Get advice on which plants are poisonous or have irritant sap.

- Be wary of trees and plants that produce berries which might fall onto the path and stain and cause confusion.

These guidelines are not exhaustive but should be sufficient to encourage people to provide a garden where at all possible.

All the recommendations made in this chapter will facilitate a calm, predictable, sensible, familiar, suitably stimulating and safe environment. They are, however, only the backdrop against which person-centred, holistic care and support should be given. The environment is more than just the bricks and mortar of the physical surroundings. It is also the milieu in which relationships are made, expectations conveyed and relationships acknowledged (Kerr 1997).

Summary

People with a learning disability and dementia, like those without dementia, are controlled and influenced by their environment. Unlike people without dementia it is very hard for people with dementia to manipulate the environment to compensate for its inadequacies. Architects, designers, service providers and staff must take responsibility for designing environments that meet basic dementia-friendly criteria. The criteria are that the environments must be calm and stress-free, predictable and familiar and make sense to the person with dementia, and be safe.

There exists substantial research and practice evidence about how these criteria can be met. Most environmental changes suggested are not expensive to implement and yet they can make dramatic differences to the quality of life for the person with dementia. They will not only improve their sense of well-being, but also make the environments safer and can prevent people being moved out of their home into unfamiliar and sometimes locked accommodation.

12

The Role of Technology

This chapter will describe some of the ways in which technology can be used to assist people with a learning disability and dementia. Much of the technology described has been developed to enable people who are fairly independent and living in their own home, usually with minimal support from outside agencies. Some of the technology can, however, be usefully applied to the homes of people living in group situations where there is more than minimal support.

Taylor (2006, p. 9) comments that 'technology can be used to ensure safety and security, operate as a memory aid, identify the person's location or alert others of care needs'. Further, 'Assistive technology can fulfil all of these roles at any given time'.

Safety and security

In the kitchen, detectors for smoke and carbon monoxide can be essential safety devices to support the continued use of the cooking area. These systems can be linked both to internal and external alarm systems and to automated window openers to remove the build-up of harmful gases.

Cookers can be set to operate only at certain times of day. The cooker can be set to go on at times when the person normally cooks meals, but to switch off at other times to prevent the risk of the cooker being left on for long periods, unattended. There are other similar devices such as a microwave that turns itself off if metal is accidentally placed in the oven.

The use of a camera door entry system can enable the person with a learning disability and dementia to allow only certain people into their home. Some people with dementia have been taught to let in only people whose face matches a photo board next to the door entry system.

Flood prevention can be critical to ensuring the person with a learning disability and dementia can remain at home. There is an increased risk that the person may forget they have started to fill a sink or bath. The person may have to be admitted to emergency care while repairs are made to their home and this may lead to their routine being so disrupted that it is difficult to reintroduce them to their home setting. A flood alert device can identify if the bath has filled too much or that water has overflowed on to the floor. Such a system can either shut off the water supply or alert someone via a pager or alarm. As with all alarm systems, audible alarms should be avoided if at all possible. For many people with dementia the sound of the alarm may well be distressing and may cause further confusion. An alternative method of reducing the risk of flood is the use of a bath plug with an integrated pressure value. The plug releases water through the main plughole when the weight of water above reaches a certain level.

Memory aids

Technology can operate in a number of ways to assist with memory. A voice prompt reminder device can be a memory aid for taking medication. An analogue bedside clock may be the most appropriate technology to remind someone of the time during the night. Digital clocks are a more modern invention and the person with a learning disability and dementia, when relying on their long-term memory, may not associate the series of numbers as a clock. They may then get out of bed to seek to find the time.

Should the person with a learning disability and dementia get up during the night, there are a number of assistive technologies that can be used to support them. The use of a passive infrared beam (PIR) near the exit to their bedroom or at the side of their bed can be used to switch on the bathroom light. This can cue the person to use the toilet, if the toilet is visible. This usually means that it needs to be en suite.

If the person is having difficulties distinguishing night and day, a PIR near the front door can illuminate a small light box within their visual field that lights up the words 'it's night-time, go back to bed' or a similar appropriate message. This equipment can be set to operate only at specified times. Experience suggests that the PIR light box messages should be varied in wording every two to three weeks to ensure the person does not just grow accustomed to the message and ignore it. For many people with a learning disability this will not be appropriate as they may never have been able to read; even if they learned to read later in life, this skill may soon disappear. Nevertheless there will be a few people for whom it will be suitable. A similar type of technology is available, which activates through the breaking of a circuit when the door is opened. One option is to have an audio message recorded by a familiar person to remind the person to put their coat on or take their keys when going out. However, caution is required with this type of technology as a disembodied voice could add to the confusion of the person with dementia.

Location tools

Location technology has been used both in the community and in care settings in the support of people with dementia (Miskelly 2004). This type of technology is often referred to as 'tagging'. The term 'tagging', with its association with the criminal justice system and the tagging of prisoners, has been considered inappropriate for the care system (McShane *et al.* 1998; Michau 1996). Whichever term is used the objective is the same; also the potential intrusion and benefits need to be weighed in the balance.

A number of devices can be used to help if the person with a learning disability and dementia is in danger of becoming lost. The example of the PIR monitor in the bedroom can be linked to a pager to alert staff or a family carer when the person gets up. This can enable quick intervention before the person leaves the premises. A pressure mat can serve the same purpose, but can cause a person to stumble if not positioned carefully. One benefit of these options is also that a carer does not disturb the person with dementia at night by opening the bedroom door to check if they are in bed. Another benefit is that if the person lives at home with their family, their carer can have a more settled sleep because they know the technology will alert them.

Other forms of location devices include wristbands or pendants that the person with dementia wears. This can set off a pager when the person exits through specific doors. This type of system is similar to those found in shops to prevent theft.

If the person does leave the house new technology can have a role to play in locating them. Attention is being given to newer mobile phones and other geographical positioning systems (GPS) that can be used to locate the person if they get lost. The system can be used simply to keep a track on the person so that after they have been out for a while they are easy to find. These will have a role to play in supporting certain individuals. These devices require that someone makes sure the person is wearing the phone, that the battery is charged and more importantly that it is switched on (Miskelly 2004).

Assistance with care

Other devices can offer an essential lifeline for the person living alone. A telephone with large pre-programmable picture buttons, behind which friends or carers' photos can be placed, can compensate for forgetting familiar numbers. This can allow the person with a learning disability to seek help easily if they require it.

An epilepsy bed monitor can be placed below the mattress to alert staff to the onset of a seizure. This can speed up the response from staff. Seizures, alongside mobility problems, can increase the risk of someone with a learning disability and dementia falling. The use of a fall monitor that is activated by the impact of the fall and the person being in a horizontal position can help. This is dependent on ensuring that the person is wearing the device.

Case study 21

Anne is a 70-year-old woman with a learning disability who has recently been diagnosed with dementia of the Alzheimer's type. Anne had moved into a six-bedded small group home eight years ago, having previously lived in a large institution. Anne has good physical health and mobility and has always enjoyed walking. When Anne lived in the institution, she spent most of her day out in the garden or walking along the many corridors in the hospital. Since Anne moved to her new home she has had a routine of walking to the local park in the morning, having her lunch at a café and then coming home in the late afternoon.

Recently, Anne has got lost when returning to her home and has had to ask for help. On two occasions the police have had to assist Anne to find her way home as she was found a number of miles away from her usual route. The staff at the home have become very concerned about the situation, especially as there are a number of busy roads nearby for Anne to cross.

To support Anne to maintain her routine, staff began to walk with her to and from the park. However, Anne did not like this, as she prefers her own company and began to ask them to stop following her. Staff began to discuss the idea of introducing a location device to help if Anne does get lost.

The home planned to have Anne carry a special type of mobile device with GPS technology. This technology would operate in such a way that Anne's journey could be tracked and her whereabouts at any given time easily identified. If this technology is to be used to support Anne, then checks also need to be in place to ensures the following questions are addressed:

- Has Anne's consent (or her representative's) been sought to use this assistive technology to support her?
- What methods of communication have been used to ensure Anne understands what is being asked of her?
- Has a date been set to review the use of this assistive technology intervention?
- What methods will be used to evaluate the effectiveness of the assistive technology in Anne's care?

The use of technology should not be considered as a separate part of an individual's care, but be integrated into the overall care planning process (Wey 2006). Technologies should be used only after detailed individual needs assessments have been done. The global application of technologies should be considered only if this would enable everyone to be equally supported. A technology that suits one person may be completely wrong for someone else. A technology that may give someone freedom may be intrusive and restrictive for someone else. It is, of course, also central to the use of the various technologies cited that there is an appropriate staff or carer response. Technology is to be used as an additional tool in the maintenance of skills, independence and dignity and not as a substitute for adequate staffing levels.

Summary

There are an increasing number of technologies being developed that can be used in group living situations. These will enable the person with dementia to be safer and potentially have an improved quality of life. The use of technologies that will alert carers to potentially dangerous situations can also assist the person with dementia to be safe without staff feeling the need constantly to check them.

13

Late and End Stage Care

Dementia is a progressive condition that will ultimately lead to death. The progress will be different for everyone but ultimately staff, carers and peers need to be prepared for the death. It is of concern that often this is not prepared for and people can be moved out of their home in the late stage, simply because of lack of forward planning that leads to a lack of adequate resources. There is no way to predict the length of time the person will survive with the condition. For people with Down's syndrome the progression appears to be quicker than for other people but this does not neccssarily mean that this will always be the case. As the condition progresses, people may be affected by illnesses, such as aspiration pneumonia as well as other infections and traumas that can have a profound impact.

These developments will probably cause the person to lose many skills and abilities. This can sometimes make it appear that they are entering the end stage. There is always a danger that the person is moved to a nursing resource when, with the use of antibiotics and other medication, they may well return completely or partly to their previous level of ability.

Case study 22

Paul was a man in his late sixties with a learning disability and a diagnosis of Alzheimer's disease. He had had the condition for many years and was clearly losing many skills. He was admitted to hospital with aspiration pneumonia. He appeared to be close to death. He was unresponsive to any stimulus; he appeared not to know where he was or who was with him. He woke for short periods but mostly he slept.

His family were contacted and staff and relatives gathered to spend what they anticipated were the last days with Paul. The pneumonia was treated successfully. Three weeks later Paul was at home, eating with everyone else, taking part in the daily activities of the house and, generally, cheerful. He did not return to the skill level he had before the episode but he was certainly very much alive.

The same occurred three more times over the next two years. Paul died after the third episode.

This case study underlines the fact there is a need to resist the temptation to believe someone is at the end stage when with correct intervention they may return to a level close the to their previous abilities.

Nevertheless the person will inevitably lose skills and abilities. It is at the later stage that staff require special knowledge, skills and sensitivity. There is a need for extra support and training. This can be a difficult time both physically and emotionally. It is often at this stage that the hope that people will remain and die at home becomes increasingly difficult to sustain.

At the late stage, the following changes will generally be experienced. The person may:

- forget how to eat and drink
- be unable to sit up
- lose the ability to maintain balance
- find walking increasingly difficult
- lose bowel and bladder control
- become significantly less active
- experience changes in their metabolism
- have substantial weight loss
- experience the loss of both short- and long-term memories
- lose their ability to recognise previously familiar people and environments
- experience seizure activity
- become bedridden
- become inactive
- be at great risk of choking and becoming dehydrated
- be at risk of developing pressure sores

- be at great risk of infection
- easily develop aspiration pneumonia
- develop hypertonia
- experience a complete loss of self-care skills.

As the condition progresses towards the end stage, the person will show little emotional response and may appear not to recognise when someone is in the room with them. It is easy at this stage to imagine that the person is oblivious to their surroundings. Of course we cannot know what is happening for them; they cannot tell us and we have to try to guess from, sometimes, slight changes in facial expression, especially changes in the expression in the eyes. Often people will appear to be frightened: it does not take much imagination to sense that they may feel alone and scared. It is important to keep talking gently to the person so that they know they are not alone. Much of the time there may be no response but often people will come, as if out of a fog, and smile in recognition and sometimes despite the almost complete lose of verbal skills people will in the late stages suddenly say something. It can be both disconcerting and rewarding at this stage when someone does speak. It is so important that someone is there and that the phrase or words are listened to. They may still respond to sensory stimulation; touch, aromatherapy and music should be used. Don't let go; the person is still there somewhere.

Case study 23

As a child, 47-year-old Jenny had attended ballet classes. Being short and plump did not stop her from carrying herself and acting as a ballet dancer and offering her hand to visitors in a royal manner. The ballet *Cinderella* was her favourite story; indeed, in the earlier stages of dementia after a visit to the ballet to see *Cinderella*, she had told her support worker that 'the prince was dancing with me … everyone was looking at me. I say to myself "I wish I was Cinderella"'. Also 'The handsome prince took my hand and said "You are beautiful sweetheart"'. Jenny's support worker recalls that in the end stages of the condition, when Jenny was very frail, confined to bed and unable to speak, 'We could raise a smile by taking her hand in the royal manner and calling her princess'.

This case study highlights, again, the importance of life story work. Without the information about Jenny's past, staff might have missed an important way to amuse and communicate with her. It also serves to underline the fact that with the right information and attention, there is still the possibility of contact and reassurance, even at the later stages when people may appear to be unaware of their surroundings.

It might be assumed that at end stage, people require less staff time and attention. They will not be so active and so staff do not have to be so attentive to the sometimes random, risky and 'challenging' behaviour that for whatever reason will have diminished. Certainly they will demand less but that does not mean that they do not need and want staff time. It is essential that, just because the person is no longer so demanding of time and attention, staff time is not automatically reduced.

At the late stage people will need one-to-one support with the provision of 24-hour support and care at the very late stage. This will also be a time of emotional stress and strain. The impact on staff, peers and relatives must be acknowledged and accommodated. Everyone will need support to cope with their grief as well as the demands of caring for someone in the terminal stages of the condition.

For relatives this can be a terrible time of mixed emotions. Many will say that the person has slowly been lost to them and they will have started grieving for the loss of the person they knew and loved earlier on in the condition. Peers may also find the changes distressing. They may find it very hard to be with their friend in the late stages. The changes can be frightening and they may need help to accept what is happening. For staff it may be the first death they have experienced amongst the people they support.

Wilkinson *et al.* (2004) recommend that the emotional strain needs to be acknowledged by giving staff shorter shifts, as the emotional toll can be high. They also recommend the employment of specialist, trained staff to support other tenants and residents, who can often feel left out by the amount of attention paid to the person who is dying.

What support and treatment need to be in place?

When people become bedridden, there is a high risk of the development of bedsores. The provision of special mattresses and regular turning are essential. Pressure sores are preventable and may indicate inadequate attention and poor care. Once the person is less mobile, advice must be sought from a pressure sore care specialist. The specialist will use a specific ratings chart to check the condition of the person's skin. Their advice must be followed diligently and without variation, and must be on the agenda of each staff handover meeting. Much of the advice will include the following:

- Change clothes regularly – sweaty clothes can cause irritation.
- If the person is confined to bed, turn them every two hours. Use a special mattress that reduces pressure areas (air mattress) for chairs, wheelchairs and beds.
- Keep bedding loose.
- Use recommended cream on pressure areas such as hips, sacrum, heels, shoulders and buttocks.
- Maintain activity levels as much as possible (active or passive movement).
- A good diet will help to keep the skin healthier and more resistant to sores.
- Pay constant attention to hydration. People should drink one and a half litres of fluid a day. Without this the skin dries and cracks easily.
- Use baby oil on skin after washing. If talcum powder is needed use sparingly.
- Use non-perfumed washing powders and fabric conditioners.
- Ensure that incontinence is dealt with appropriately. This will require ongoing assessment of appropriate incontinence aids.
- Ensure that urine and faeces do not remain in contact with the skin.
- Avoid tight and uncomfortable clothing.
- Ensure that there are no rough seams in clothing.

- Check that no objects are left in pockets as these can cause friction.

- Ensure that people are thoroughly dried after bathing, particularly in the skin folds. Under breasts, groin and underarms need special attention. Pat rather than rub dry.

- Always seek reassessment and ongoing support from the community or palliative care nurse. Ask the specialist nurse for a monitoring chart and complete regularly.

The lack of activity will also often lead to an increased risk of infection, especially pneumonia. Advice and guidance from a physiotherapist and an occupational therapist will be critical at this stage.

Because eating becomes a problem, the advice of a speech and language therapist is essential. The importance of using the correct food and making sure that the person is sitting properly to try to avoid choking become paramount at this stage. It may be necessary to consider the use of percutaneous endoscopic gastrostomy (PEG feeding); this is dealt with in more detail in Chapter 10 on supporting people to eat well.

It should be a constant concern that people may be in pain and not able to communicate this. The local hospice should be asked for advice and guidance. Research shows that at this stage, staff require some assistance from a palliative care nurse but that there is no automatic need for people to go into the hospice (Wilkinson *et al.* 2004).

Summary

Dementia is a terminal condition. It is crucial that service providers antici-pate the needs of the person at the later and end stages. Without resources being put in place in time, the person may be moved unnecessarily. Input from specialist professionals, a speech and language therapist, a skin care specialist, an occupational therapist and a palliative care nurse must be sought.

People will not be so demanding of staff, because of a reduction in risky, unexpected and perhaps 'challenging' behaviour. This should not lead to an assumption that less staff time is needed. People may not demand the attention but at this stage they need the constant reassurance of the presence of staff. The need to provide this and to provide the increased physical care, such as turning the person every two hours, has an impact on other tenants and residents, who may feel neglected and who themselves may require more staff time than is often available.

The grief and stress experienced by relatives, peers and staff at this stage should be acknowledged and they must be given support and attention.

Issues and Concerns for Relatives

Case study 24

Maureen's younger brother Ross had Down's syndrome. Maureen had always been very close to him and had promised their mother that, when she died, Maureen would continue to care for him. After their mother's death Ross moved in with his sister.

At the age of 49 Ross developed Alzheimer's type dementia. Maureen continued to look after him but her own health began to fail as Ross became more disabled and demanding of her time. Maureen refused all offers of help. She wanted to honour the promise she had given to her mother and she was worried that no one else would love and care for her brother as she did. Only when the situation was at breaking point was Ross given a place in a small residential house. His sister felt that she had been a complete failure.

Maureen was left in an emotional turmoil with mixed and confusing feelings towards the staff. On the one hand she felt enormous gratitude towards the staff at the home; on the other hand she had a constant nagging doubt about their care and worried that they did not give Ross sufficient care and love. Her worries and anxieties were exacerbated by the changes she saw in Ross. His deteriorating condition made her anxious that this may be because of the lack of staff time and attention rather than the inevitable consequence of the condition.

It might be that someone comes into the care of the services after living with a family member who is no longer able to cope as the condition progresses. This is potentially more traumatic for the relative than in cases where their sibling or adult child has already been supported elsewhere. The sense of failure and guilt at no longer being able to cope can be overwhelming. It can lead to relatives not visiting because of their painful feelings. It is important that staff recognise this and make it as easy as possible for the relative to visit. Acknowledge with them how hard it is and encourage them to remain as involved as possible in the care and decision making. Staff need to be aware that their competence, whilst at one level welcome, can feel like a rebuke to the relative who is no longer able to cope.

Family members, such as Maureen, will have known the person with dementia all of their lives. They will know more about them and in particular about their history, probably, than anyone else. They will remember behaviours and habits that the person had as a child, teenager and young adult. The return of these behaviours as the dementia progresses may be new and inexplicable to staff but the knowledge of siblings can help to explain and fill the gap. This, yet again, underlines the importance of undertaking life story work. More information on this can be found in Chapter 6 on therapeutic interventions.

Often it is the relatives who are able to fight for services when staff are restricted. The role of sisters as advocates is well documented in the publications *Caring for Kathleen* (Fray 2000) and *An Example of Good Practice* (Lewis 2003). These are vivid testimony to the critical role played by relatives, and in these two cases by sisters, fighting for good practice. The drive and passion evidenced in these publications is replicated amongst other relatives. It should not be squandered or ignored.

There will be varying levels of family involvement with the person with dementia. If the person has been in residential care or supported living, relatives may no longer live close by. This does not mean that they are not involved. Whatever the level of involvement it is critical that staff capitalise on this. They need to be proactive in encouraging, supporting and valuing the contributions of relatives. It is important to keep relatives well informed of all developments and to seek their involvement, as appropriate, in decision making.

Relatives will often find it hard to come to terms with the fact that their son, daughter, sister or brother has dementia. Initially there may be an element of denial; other reasons for the changes in behaviour may be given. As the person's condition deteriorates, the sense of loss of the person they knew will mean that people will begin to grieve. This grieving may involve anger that can be directed towards staff. Staff will need to understand this as part of grieving and use supervision and support to enable them to cope.

It seems to many a cruel fate that brings another disability on top of the one already present. Many relatives will have fought all their lives to get the service they have for their relative and are fearful that this will be lost because of the onset of the dementia.

As part of a research project I had this anxiety expressed to me thus:

> I suppose in a way I would be scared to ask them what's going to happen, because they could say he might be moved into hospital.

> I wouldn't like him to go anywhere else because I don't think he will get as good a place as this. He is settled. (Wilkinson *et al.* 2004, p.21)

It is critical that relatives are given specific information about their relative with dementia. They should also be given the opportunity to attend any course offered to staff. However, relatives have indicated that they want access to leaflets or books and an opportunity to talk to someone about the condition rather than attend courses (Wilkinson *et al.* 2004).

Relatives will often have scant information about dementia. Their lack of understanding about the impact of the condition on their relative and how to best interact with them means that they are often left exacerbating challenging situations and feeling confused, powerless and fearful.

The lack of knowledge about the condition is illustrated well by the following questions that I have been asked by relatives:

> Is it part of the brain that is dying off?

> Why did he get so agitated?

> Why were the stairs difficult?

> He had problems seeing how to go, why was that? (Wilkinson *et al.* 2004, p. 21)

It is of concern that, often, relatives are not told that the condition is terminal. This is a painful thing to have to acknowledge and the temptation to avoid it is perhaps great but it must be overcome. Relatives need to know what to prepare for and to begin to come to terms with the inevitable outcome. As death approaches, relatives will need more support and to be given the opportunity to spend time with their relative and to be there at the end.

There are a few relatives who, having been barely involved with the care of the person with dementia, will want to be involved at the end, particularly with funeral arrangements. Staff understandably can feel resentful of this when they have been the main carers and are themselves grieving and needing to have the type of funeral that will help them come to terms with their loss. This is a less common scenario than the one where family and staff have worked together and can plan a joint funeral that meets the needs of everyone involved.

Summary

Relatives will often have great difficulty accepting that they can no longer provide the level of care and support that the person with dementia requires. The point at which this is acknowledged is often when the carer is at breaking point. Staff need to be sensitive to the needs of carers in this position. They will need reassurance that staff understand and are aware of the feelings of guilt and failure that can underlie complaints about the level of care that the person with dementia is being given.

Relatives must be, where possible and appropriate, included in the care of and decision making about the person. Staff need to be proactive in engaging them. The relative will often have known the person with dementia for all of their lives and will have vital information, which will help staff to understand the person's changing behaviours as the condition progresses.

Relatives, however, often have very little knowledge about dementia and should be given advice and information that will help them understand the changes that are taking place in the person with dementia. This will also help them to understand the impact of their own interactions with the person with dementia.

Dementia is a terminal condition. Relatives are often not made aware of this, or can, through denial, block the acknowledgement of this fact. Staff must work with them to help them and include them in preparations for the death and funeral.

15

Some Issues in Relation to Medication

It is not within the remit of this book to present detailed information on medication, its uses, impact and efficacy. It is important, however, that people supporting and providing services for those with a learning disability know some of the key issues in relation to medication as they relate to people with a learning disability and dementia. This knowledge should enable them to be better informed about the consequences of the use of some medications and should also enable them to discuss some of their concerns about the use of various medications and methods of taking drugs.

Many people with a learning disability will have been on medication for all or most of their lives. The use of anticonvulsants for epilepsy and medication for diabetes and hypothyroidism particularly amongst people with Down's syndrome is more common (Selby 2001), but there will be many other drugs that people will have been taking for a long time. The onset of the conditions of older age will often result in the use of additional drugs. This increase in the level of drug taking (polypharmacy) can lead to serious side effects and even the onset of an acute confusional state or delirium. It is essential therefore that staff are aware of changes that may be the result of an increase in the number or type of medication being pre-scribed. Staff must be willing and able to bring these to the notice of the medical practitioner involved. Medications need to be reviewed on a regular basis to avoid the unwanted side effects of drug interactions (Livingston 2003). It is also important to be aware that because of the changes in our metabolism that occur with ageing, drugs that people have previously tolerated well may begin to have adverse side effects. It is important not to assume that the problems with tolerance are simply related to recently prescribed medication. The person may be reacting to something that they have previously and for a long time been able to take safely.

The use of neuroleptic (antipsychotic) medication

The use of neuroleptic drugs, also referred to as 'major tranquillisers' and 'antipsychotic' medication, needs to be addressed. These drugs, often used for their sedative affect, can cause further cognitive deterioration and confusion; some will induce akathisia. (Akathisia is a frequent and common adverse effect of treatment with neuroleptic drugs. It can cause feelings of restlessness and make the person feel they need to move. The person may also rock while standing or sitting, and lift their feet as if marching on the spot and cross and uncross their legs while sitting.) They can also cause drug-induced Parkinsonism. This may then require further medication to compensate for the effects of the primary drug. It is important, therefore, that there is a 'careful appraisal of the person's whole situation and the likely balance between overall benefit and adversity to the individual' (Hopker 1999, p. 108) before these drugs are used.

Robertson *et al.* (2000) found that there were high levels of prescription for neuroleptic drugs for people with dementia. This may well be replicated amongst people with a learning disability and dementia.

If, after a thorough assessment, the use of neuroleptic medication is necessary, it is imperative that it forms part of a clear treatment plan (Deb, Clarke and Unwin 2006; Scottish Intercollegiate Guidelines Network (SIGN) 1986) and that the National Institute for Health and Clinical Excellence (NICE 2006) and SIGN guidelines are adhered to.

Methods of taking medication

The size and shape of the tablet can be an issue as the person with a learning disability and dementia may have been given medication in the past that was large and hard to swallow. Although considerable effort has been made by the pharmaceutical industry to make tablets smaller and easier to swallow, the person may be resistant to taking any form of tablet.

The memory of past difficulties in relation to taking medication may lead to renewed anxiety particularly in relation to swallowing tablets. The taking of medication may also be associated with other negative experiences, such as having to take a tablet because the person was unable to manage their behaviour.

As part of the assessment for medication, it is important to find out about the person's history and preference in taking medication. Often the medication section of an assessment form is seen as something that the doctor or nurse completes and is only to be used to state the types of medication the person is currently on. However, further information needs to be recorded to inform carers and clinicians of the person's other needs relating to the taking of medication. The person may have a preference for taking medication in a liquid form, or they may have a dislike for tablets that dissolve. They may have preferences or routines that help them take medication, for example the person may like to take their tablets with a particular drink.

It may be that as the condition progresses, and people return to past habits, old routines will need to be reinstated. For example, people may in the past have developed particular routines that staff or parents instigated to facilitate the taking of medication. Consider the example of a woman with a learning disability and dementia who used to take her inhaler after someone counted from one to three. Although this had ceased as a prompt in her later years, it had returned as a prerequisite when dementia made her reality that of her younger years.

The way in which a medication is given must at all times follow pharmaceutical manufacturers' and clinical guidelines. For example, certain tablet medications should not be crushed or taken with other medications (Wright *et al.* 2006). The crushing of medication should always be avoided unless it is specifically stated that this is an acceptable way to administer a drug. The crushing of medication can significantly alter its efficacy. If a person has specific swallowing difficulties or they receive their medication through a tube, then clinical guidance on this should be followed thoroughly. It is often necessary to employ alternative means of giving medication than simply giving tablets. The use of liquid medication, medication that dissolves under the tongue and a transdermal patch may provide a useful range of options to help the person receive the right treatment in the right dose with the least disruption.

Cholinesterase inhibitors

Cholinesterase inhibitors, sometimes called 'cognitive enhancers', work by reducing the loss of acetylcholine in the brain. It is thought that it is the loss of this chemical that leads to a decline in cognitive function and attendant short-term memory loss, loss of verbal memory, recognition, orientation and self-awareness and consequent related behavioural changes. There are three cholinesterase inhibiting drugs:

- donepezil (Aricept)
- rivastigmine (Exelon)
- galatamine (Reminyl).

The use of these drugs can improve cognitive function and behavioural changes (Birks 2005). They do not slow down the progression of the condition and will not alter the time of death. They may, however, give the person with dementia an improved quality of life.

The decision to prescribe or continue with administration needs to take account of some of the more common side effects such as:

- urinary incontinence
- convulsions
- diarrhoea
- nausea
- loss of appetite.

Case study 25

Andrew, a man with Down's syndrome, was diagnosed with dementia at the age of 49 years. Andrew became increasingly disorientated and distressed. He began to lose many of the skills of daily living and was in need of much more support. At the request of the family, the clinical psychologist approached the consultant psychiatrist and GP to prescribe Aricept.

Once the correct dosage was achieved (at one stage too high a dose was given with consequent side effects), this led to a dramatic improvement in Andrew's capacity and abilities. Andrew regained lost skills and comprehension and just as importantly he regained his 'zest and enthusiasm for life'. He was even able to travel by plane to visit his sisters. After nine months the impact of the drug began to diminish and Andrew was taken off Aricept. His decline was then sudden and rapid. The use of the drug had, however, provided wonderful gains and opportunities for Andrew and all concerned with his care and support. The nine months that he was on the drug gave the organisation providing his care time to get everything in place for him. One-to-one support, housing adaptations and staff training meant that when Andrew came off the drug the social, emotional and physical environment was in place to provide him with the best care and support. The nine months gave Andrew time to enjoy an improved quality of life. It also gave his family more time to enjoy him as he had always been.

(Adapted from Lewis 2003)

There has been little systematic research into the benefits of the various cholinesterase inhibiting drugs on people with a learning disability and dementia. Prasher (2005) conducted a small study on the use of Rivagstimine, however, and concluded that people with Down's syndrome and dementia of the Alzheimer's type 'would benefit from treatment with' this drug.

There is, at the time of writing, considerable debate around the use of cholinesterase inhibitors. NICE have stated that these can now be provided only at mid-stage dementia. Previously the drugs were given at the early stage with, as in the case of Andrew described above, sometimes dramatic but often simply worthwhile benefits. Although there is need for further study it does already appear to be the case that some people with a learning disability and dementia would benefit from the use of these drugs. Indeed the NICE guidelines published in November 2006 make a point of singling out people with a learning disability for a different approach to the prescription of the cholinesterase inhibitors. The NICE committee considered that people with a learning disability fall into a subgroup of people who would benefit considerably more from the use of the cholinesterase inhibitors than others and that, for this subgroup, 'it might be a relatively cost effective treatment' (NICE 2006, p. 45). The committee considered that 'The interests of learning disability patients were best served by including initiation of treatment by learning disability specialists' and, further, 'the committee felt that learning disability specialists were best placed to judge entry and continuation criteria for people with a learning disability' (NICE 2006, p. 47). Perhaps people with a learning disability will find that they are prescribed these drugs when they are being denied to the general population with dementia.

Summary

As people age their metabolism changes. They may develop adverse responses to drugs that they have previously tolerated. They may also have adverse responses to drug combinations and the effects of polypharmacy. Neuroleptic (antipsychotic) medication has a role to play but it can have serious side effects. It should, therefore, be undertaken only when other possible responses have been considered and eliminated.

Cholinesterase inhibitors can have an important role in mitigating some of the adverse effects of the condition, particularly in the early stages. The recommendations of the NICE (2006) report are that specialist learning disability professionals should be the people charged with making decisions about the use of these drugs for people with a learning disability and dementia.

Models of Care

The model of care that informs a service will determine the type and range of solutions offered to people as their dementia and needs change. The type, level and location of the support and provision given to the person will determine whether someone stays at home or is moved. It will also determine where they are moved to, when they are moved and how this is implemented. The philosophy of care and the resources available that underpin these decisions do not exist in a vacuum. They are the consequence of knowledge, decisions and commitment within the service. The resources available are determined, of course, to some extent by budgetary restraints but they are also a manifestation of a philosophy of care.

This chapter will outline the models of service delivery that are available to service providers and will address the implications of each model for people with dementia, peers and staff. This includes the implications and considerations involved in moving someone out of their home. The models used and outlined below are based on those described by Janicki and Dalton (1998) and Wilkinson *et al.* (2004).

The four models described are:

- ageing in place
- in place progression
- referral out
- outreach.

Ageing in place

In the 'ageing in place' model every possible effort is made to enable the person to continue to live (and die) in their own home, so the service makes constant adaptations to the accommodation – the home – of the person to meet their changing needs. These adaptations will involve the implementation of much that is contained in this book, including the training of staff in dementia care, the making of adaptations to the built environment and work with other residents and tenants who live with the person. There would also be an increased use of and developed relationship with other professionals such as speech and language therapists, incontinence advisers and palliative care nurses, who would be used in the support package.

It is probably the case that most people involved in supporting people with a learning disability and dementia would choose the 'ageing in place' option. This is the preferred option because it means that the person will be surrounded by familiar people in a familiar environment. Their carers and peers will be better placed than anyone else to understand them and will often have close emotional ties that enable them to cope with changing and increasing demands. This route, however, is often not an option for a number of reasons.

Case study 26

Diane is a 72-year-old woman with a learning disability and dementia. Diane had lived with two other women in her supported house for eight years. The house was a Victorian three-bedroomed semi-detached. All the bedrooms were upstairs and there was no room downstairs to convert into a bedroom. Diane was no longer safe to use the stairs. The use of a stair lift would have been terrifying for her.

Diane and the other two women in the house had always fiercely guarded their independence and resented anything other than minimal intervention and support. As Diane's dementia progressed, more and more people were involved in her support. Her night-time disturbance and daytime confusion necessitated waking night staff and 24-hour support on site. The quality of life for the other two women was being seriously impaired by what they experienced as an increasing intrusion and lack of privacy. They increasingly expressed their resentment.

In recognition of the fact that this situation was going to get worse, a decision was made to move Diane to a resource with no stairs and where her care would not intrude on the lives of others.

This case study is an example of where 'ageing in place' is not a practicable, viable option. It highlights a common reason for people being moved from their home. The lack of downstairs sleeping accommodation and toilet often means that the house becomes unsafe for the person with dementia. Problems with depth perception and decreasing mobility can leave the person trapped upstairs. It is essential that service planners take note of the needs of an ageing learning disabled population who, with or without dementia, are going to be increasingly disabled by stairs.

The reaction of other people in the house can also be critical in determining whether the person with dementia stays or goes. Diane's housemates were experiencing a number of intrusive changes in their own lives. The needs of the people without dementia have to be weighed against those of the person with dementia and the latter may, as a consequence, need to be removed from the situation. I have had the experience of residents and tenants who live with a person with dementia expressing feelings of annoyance and loss because the person with dementia is getting more attention. They feel that as a consequence they are losing out. One woman expressed this thus: 'My key worker spends so much time with Pete she does not have time for me; I think Pete should be somewhere else'. When she was asked where she would want to live if she had dementia, this woman and her other housemates replied unequivocally that they would not want to be moved. This is a dilemma that providers need to address.

This problem can sometimes be alleviated if there are adequate increased resources, for example an increase in staffing levels. However, this is not always achieved or achievable. This is substantially because services have not been 'dementia ready' but have waited until after someone has been given a diagnosis of dementia before beginning to put dementia-friendly design features and staff training in place. After the diagnosis has been made, there needs to be an allocation of a pot of money that can be drawn on quickly to pay for the various resources that will need to be allocated at various stages, as the dementia progresses and the person's needs change. Staff should not have to keep applying on an ad-hoc basis for new resources to meet the changing needs of the person. If this allocation is not done, the resource acquisition, be it of one-to-one support, extra hours cover, waking night staff or new equipment, lags behind need. Often by the time the new resource has been allocated, it no longer meets the changed needs of the person with dementia.

Sometimes even with the allocation of increased staffing and the implementation of adaptations to the building, the necessary level of care cannot be given and the person has to move. This is particularly the case when the person requires nursing care that either is not available or has not been accessed within the learning disability service.

'In place progression'

In the 'in place progression' model the learning disability service provides a specialist resource for people with dementia. In its most pure form this service would be a distinct and separate building and resource with all the dementia-friendly building design features discussed in Chapter 11 on the environment. The staff would have a high level of expertise and knowledge about both dementia and learning disability. This service could also provide expertise and resources to 'ageing in place' providers.

The use of the 'in place progression' model can address many of the problems indicated above. Below is an example of such a service model in practice.

Oldham Social Services 'in place progression' provision

This resource was established, within the learning disability service, in response to the changing needs of people with a learning disability who had dementia living in the locality. The decision to fund the project was driven by the recognition that, without it, people would continue to be moved into nursing home provision for older people. This had been the practice up to this point. This had proved to be detrimental to both their health and their well-being.

The house was set up to provide for four people with dementia on the ground floor. It was designed to provide a calm, predictable and failure-free environment in which both health and social needs are met.

Staff were given the option to say whether or not they would like to work with this client group. The staff, all social care staff, were trained in dysphagia, the use of suction, positioning, manual handling, pressure area care and postural drainage. They were also given person-centred, dementia-specific training. An adviser in best practice in this type of provision was identified and used to inform the service development.

Staffing levels are higher than elsewhere in the service. Waking night staff were employed to accommodate the needs of people waking, who might need turning or to be supported to eat at night.

A good working relationship was established with the local GP practice. The GPs work to keep people at home; they attend best practice meetings and are alert to the fact that, when people are near death, they need to notify the out-of-hours service so that admission to hospital occurs only if absolutely necessary. Contact was maintained with other service users and staff who knew the people before they moved into the house.

Significantly this provision has become a resource for other providers. The expertise developed is now used to advise others. This has further enabled people to remain in their own homes for as long as possible. It is important to note that this service is embedded within a wider provision of resources with trained and knowledgeable staff. Such provision cannot stand alone.

As in the example given, an 'in place progression' model can facilitate the continuation of contact with familiar staff and peers. It also provides highly trained staff and an appropriate physical environment. It can also enable the development of expertise amongst other professionals who are involved with this model. Wilkinson *et al.* (2004) found that where this model existed, the doctors in the local medical centre had also developed expertise and interest in this patient group. Of course if someone needs hospitalisation, then there is no argument, but it is important to determine if, with the right resource, they could remain within the learning disability service with staff who know about their specific needs.

This model can provide an ideal alternative to the 'ageing in place' model. It is, however, not without its own potential disadvantages and problems. It does involve moving people and so they lose their home. The place may also, at times, be full when someone else needs the resource. Conversely there will be times when it is underused by people with dementia. This can leave empty beds, which need to be filled. Sometimes, because of the high cost of this provision and the presence of well-trained staff, this can lead to pressure for other people with complex needs to be accommodated. This can mean that people who are particularly noisy and 'challenging' are moved into an environment that needs to be calm and stress-free.

It can also mean that staff working in the unit are always working with people at the later stages of the condition and so they experience people dying much more than they would normally. This can place strain on them and may lead to higher rates of staff illness and stress.

'Referral out'

The 'referral out' model involves the person being removed from the learning disability service and placed into older people's services. This usually involves a move to a nursing care home for older people. This move is usually made when the changing needs of the person can no longer be met within the learning disability service. A frequent reason for people moving out of their supported, residential or parents' home is because of their need for nursing care. It is undoubtedly true that people will sometimes need to be moved to hospital or nursing home care to receive the level of nursing and medical intervention they require.

There are nursing care homes that provide excellent medical and social care and where the person with a learning disability and dementia will experience an appropriate and person-centred service. This cannot, however, be assumed to be the norm; care managers, doctors and others responsible for making the decision to move someone must be aware of the nature of the service being provided.

There are a number of reasons why the 'referral out' model should be used with extreme caution. Staff in older people's services will often express anxiety about caring for people with a learning disability and will, often through fear and lack of knowledge and experience, fail to give adequate care (Thompson and Wright 2001; Wilkinson *et al.* 2004).

When a decision has been made to move someone, it is essential that there are clear benefits to the person. To move someone into a nursing home because there are nursing staff available but where the person may not receive adequate care in other areas such as eating, washing and skin care (Wilkinson *et al.* 2004) is questionable. The balance of gains and losses needs to be given considered, multidisciplinary and well-informed consideration.

It is not enough to simply move someone because a nursing home has had people with learning disability before. Without knowledge about how they fared, what the staff know about dementia and, importantly, what their experience and knowledge is of people with a learning disability, this is not a well-informed decision. Placing people with a learning disability, who may be in their forties and fifties if they have Down's syndrome, with older people without a learning disability, who may be in their late seventies and eighties, is inappropriate in terms of meeting individual assessed needs. People with a learning disability will often have had different life experiences to the general population and these need to be reflected in the activities and interactions that occur.

It is also the case that people are often moved because they require a level of nursing care that could and should be provided by the district nurse, the palliative care nurse and/or the staff themselves, often with advice and support from a nurse.

'Outreach'

The 'outreach' model would use resources external to the home. It would be a coordinated service, which would provide additional support, advice and assistance to people within their own home. It could be a virtual centre that contained elements of the various resources needed by the other models. It could also be located within the 'in place progression' model, where the development of a centre of expertise and high resources could provide services to other providers. This model could exist and be managed within either the statutory, voluntary or private sector.

Moving someone to another setting

The decision to move someone to another setting is problematic. The move must be made with careful consideration of the person's needs, and with great attention paid not only to where the person moves but also to when and how this is managed. Any move is likely to cause increased confusion and agitation for the person with dementia. The need to maintain familiarity and reduce stress, as far as possible, should inform the timing and nature of the move.

An abrupt and poorly managed move can result in terrible stress for the person with dementia, peers and staff. It can also mean that peers and staff lose contact with the person. Indeed it will be highly likely to have a detrimental effect on everybody involved in the situation unless great care is taken.

When a move is made it is critical that contact with everyone of significance to the person with dementia is encouraged, and friends in particular are enabled, to maintain contact. It is also vitally important that the staff in the new setting have as much information about the person as possible. This will enable them to see beyond the dementia and see the person they are caring for as complex, with a history and a life lived. This process will be greatly facilitated through the use of life story work (see Chapter 6 on therapeutic interventions).

The suggestion that it is better to move people at the late stage 'because they will not know where they are' needs to be challenged. We do not know how much awareness people have. We do know that, even at the very end stage, people will respond to familiar voices and music and may even, after months of silence, speak. Equal attention should, therefore, be given to where and how a person at the end stage is moved.

It is unfortunate that people often move abruptly, either because of a crisis for them or sadly because a place becomes available in another setting and there is pressure to use it before it is used by someone else. This is not acceptable and the good practice of moving people only after multidisciplinary, well-informed, person-centred assessment should be maintained.

Summary

Decisions about whether, where and when to move people with a learning disability and dementia will depend on the philosophy of care of and resources available to service providers. The advantages and disadvantages of some models of care, 'ageing in place', 'in place progression', 'referral out' or 'outreach' are evaluated.

Whilst most people would probably argue for the 'ageing in place' model, this is not always suitable and does not necessarily meet everyone's needs. The decision to provide an 'in place progression' model can enable people to stay within the learning disability service, with staff who know them well and understand the needs of people with a learning disability and with dementia. With the right building and staffing the person's social, emotional, physical and health needs can be met. The decision to use a 'referral out' model, where the person will move into older people's services, can be a positive experience, but this is not generally the case. Staff in this service are usually unfamiliar with people with a learning disability and the person is often residing with people who are older and who have a different history. If staff within this service receive good quality training in learning disability and dementia, some of the obstacles may be diminished. The decision to move someone from one setting to another should be based on clear multidisciplinary, person-centred, well-informed assessment. Abrupt moves should be avoided unless absolutely necessary. Whatever the nature of the move, contact with family, staff and friends should be maintained.

A Plea for The Future

The good news is that people with a learning disability are living longer. The bad news is that their needs are in danger of being misunderstood, overlooked, or poorly met. This is particularly the case in relation to those people with a learning disability who develop dementia. Whilst there is some excellent work going on around the country, there is insufficient attention being given to the development of good services to meet the needs of this group of people.

When people like Michael, quoted in Chapter 9, state, 'Kate had Down's syndrome and she got dementia; Robert had Down's syndrome and he got dementia; Margaret has Down's syndrome and she has dementia; I have Down's syndrome', we must be truthful and say, 'Yes, you are at risk of developing the condition'. But can we say, with as much confidence, that if you do get dementia you will be provided with a level of care and support for both your social and health needs that will make the experience as emotionally and physically pain free as possible? Can we provide positive interventions that will help to maintain skills as long as possible, will enable Michael to remain at home and to continue to use his day service as long as he wants and needs to? If he does need to be moved from his home, will he be provided with state of the art buildings with highly trained dedicated staff that form part of a community-based network of care and support? If he is moved into older people's services then let it be because that service is known to provide the best and most appropriate care for his current assessed needs: the staff are familiar with the needs of older people who have a learning disability and in particular are aware of and knowledgeable about the needs of people with a learning disability who also have dementia.

Much that is written about in this book is not complicated; it is not expensive. In fact much is free or cheap to implement. It should not, therefore, be beyond the capacity of those who fund and provide services to people with a learning disability to maintain all the gains made for people with a learning disability since the 1980s, as they enter older age and perhaps develop dementia. There is an urgent need to train staff to support this group of people who have highly complex and changing needs, and to provide coherent, consistent practice based on a philosophy and models of provision that continue to be based on person-centred care. I hope this book is a contribution to those goals.

References

Alzheimer's Disease Society (1995) *Dementia in the Community, Management Strategies for General Practice.* Stirling: Dementia Services Development Centre, University of Stirling.

Antonangeli, J. (1995) *Of Two Minds.* Everett, MA: Fidelity Press.

Archibald, C. (2003) *People with Dementia in Acute Hospital Settings: A Practice Guide for Nurses.* Stirling: Dementia Services Development Centre, University of Stirling.

Ball, S., Holland, T., Huppelt, F.A., Treppner, P. and Dodd, K. (2006) *CAMDEX-DS: The Cambridge Examination for Mental Disorders of Older People with Down's Syndrome and Others with Intellectual Disabilities.* Cambridge: Cambridge University Press.

Ballard, C.G., O'Brien, J.T., Reichelt, K. and Perry, E. (2002) 'Aromatherapy as a safe and effective treatment for the management of agitation in severe dementia: the results of a double-blind, placebo-controlled trial with Melissa.' *Journal of Clinical Psychiatry 63*, 553–558.

Barber, R., Panikkar, A. and McKeith, I.G. (2001) 'Dementia with Lewy bodies: Diagnosis and management.' *International Journal of Geriatric Psychiatry 16*, Supplement 1 S12–S15.

Birks, J. (2005) 'Cholinesterase inhibitors for Alzheimer's Disease.' *Cochrane Database of Systematic Reviews* (CD005593).

Brawley, E.C. (1997) *Designing for Alzheimer's Disease.* New York: John Wiley.

Breteler, M.M.B., Claus, J.J., Van Duijn, C.M., Luner, L.J. and Hofman, A. (1992) 'Epidemiology of Alzheimer's disease.' *Epidemiologic Reviews 14*, 1, 59–82.

Buchbauer, G., Jirovitz, L. and Jager, W. (1993) 'Fragrance compounds and essential oils with sedative effects upon inhalation.' *Journal of Pharmacological Science 82*, 660–664

Buijssen, H. (2005) *The Simplicity of Dementia.* London: Jessica Kingsley Publishers.

Burgener, S.C., Jirovec, M., Murrell, L. and Barton, D. (1992) 'Caregivers and environmental variables related to difficult behaviors in institutionalized demented elderly persons.' *Journal of Gerontology: Psychology Sciences 47*, 242–249.

Burns, A., Howard, R. and Pettit, W. (1997) *Alzheimer's Disease: A Medical Companion.* Oxford: Blackwell Science.

Burns, A., Byrne, J., Ballard, C. and Holmes, C. (2002) 'Sensory stimulation in dementia.' *British Medical Journal 325*, 1312–1313.

Cairns, D. and Kerr, D. (1994) *Different Realities: A Training Guide for People with Down's Syndrome and Alzheimer's Disease.* Stirling: Dementia Services Development Centre, University of Stirling.

Calkins, M.P. (1988) *Design for Dementia: Planning Environments for the Elderly and the Confused.* Owing Mills, MD: National Health Publishing.

Cantley, C. and Wilson, R.C. (2003) *Put Yourself in my Place: Designing and Managing Care Homes for People with Dementia.* Bristol: Policy Press.

Center, J., Beange, H. and McElduff, A. (1998) 'People with mental retardation have an increased prevalence of osteoporosis: A population study.' *American Journal on Mental Retardation 103*, 19–28.

Chapman, A., Jacques, A. and Marshall, M. (1994) *Dementia Care: A Handbook for Residential and Day Care.* London: Age Concern England.

Cheston, R. and Bender, B. (1999) *Understanding Dementia: The Man with the Worried Eyes.* London: Jessica Kingsley Publishers.

Clair, A.A. (1996) *The Therapeutic Uses of Music with Older Adults.* Baltimore, MD: Health Professions Press.

Cohen, U. Day, K. (1993) *Contemporary Environments for People with Dementia.* Baltimore, MD: John Hopkins University Press.

Cohen, U. and Weisman G.D. (1991) *Holding on to Home: Designing Environments for People with Dementia.* Baltimore, MD: John Hopkins University Press.

Cohen-Mansfield, J., Werner, P. and Marx, M. (1990) 'Screaming in nursing home residents.' *Journal of American Geriatric Society 38*, 785–792.

Cooper, S-A. (1997) 'High prevalence of dementia amongst people with learning disabilities not attributed to Down's syndrome.' *Psychological Medicine 27*, 609–616.

Cooper, S-A. (1998) 'Clinical study of the effects of age on the physical health of adults with mental retardation.' *American Journal of Mental Retardation 102*, 582–589.

Cooper, S-A. (1999) 'Dementia and Learning Disabilities of Causes other then Down's Syndrome.' In S. Cox and J. Keady (eds) *Younger People with Dementia: Planning, Practice and Development.* London: Jessica Kingsley Publishers.

Cooper, S-A. and Bailey, N.M. (2001) 'Psychiatric disorders amongst adults with learning disabilities: Prevalence and relationship to ability level.' *Irish Journal of Psychological Medicine 18*, 45–53.

Cumella, S., Ransford, N., Lyons, J. and Burnham, H. (2000) 'Needs for oral care among people with an intellectual disability not in contact with community dental services.' *Journal of Intellectual Disability Research 44*, 1, 45–52.

Dawson, P. (1998) 'Cognitively impaired residents receive less pain medication than non-cognitively impaired residents.' *Perspectives 22*, 4, 16–17.

Deb, S., Clarke, D. and Unwin, G. (2006) *Using Medication to Manage Behaviour Problems among Adults with a Learning Disability.* London: Mencap.

Del Ser, T., McKeith, I., Anand, R., Cicin-Sain, A., Ferrara, R. Spiegel, R. (2000) 'Dementia with Lewy bodies: Findings from an international multicentre study.' *International Journal of Geriatric Psychiatry 15*, 11, 1034–1045.

Dodd, K., Kerr, D. and Fern, S. (2006) *Down's Syndrome and Dementia: Workbook for Staff.* Teddington: Down's Syndrome Association.

Dodd, K., Turk, V. and Christmas, M. (2005) *About Dementia: For People with Learning Disabilities.* Kidderminster: British Institute of Learning Disabilities.

Earnshaw, K. and Donnelly, V. (2001) 'Partnerships in practice.' *Learning Disability Practice 4*, 3, 27.

Evenhuis, H.M. (1995) 'Medical aspects of ageing in a population with intellectual disability: Visual impairment.' *Journal of Intellectual Disability Research 39*, 19–26.

Evenhuis, H.M. (1997) 'The natural history of dementia in ageing people with intellectual disability.' *Journal of Intellectual Disability Research 41*, 92–96.

Feil, N. (1992) *V/F Validation: The Feil Method* (2nd edition). Baltimore, MD: Health Professions Press.

Ford, G. (1996) 'Putting feeding back into the hands of the patient.' *Journal of Psychosocial Nursing and Mental Health Services 34*, 35–39.

Fransman, D. (2005) 'Can removal of back teeth contribute to chronic earwax obstruction?' *British Journal of Learning Disabilities 34*, 1, 34–41.

Fray, M.T. (2000) *Caring for Kathleen.* Kidderminster: British Institute of Learning Disabilities.

Gibson, F. (2006) *Reminiscence and Recall* (3rd edition). London: Age Concern England.

Glasgow University Affiliated Department (2002) *Primary Care Liaison Team Interim Report: Preliminary Outcomes. Report to the Glasgow Learning Disability Partnership.* Glasgow: Glasgow University Affiliated Department.

Goldsmith, M. (1996) *Hearing The Voice of people with Dementia – Opportunities and Obstacles.* London: Jessica Kingsley Publishers.

Gotell, E. (2003) 'Singing, background music and music-events in the communication between persons with dementia and their caregivers.' Thesis, Blekinge Institute of Technology, Sweden: Karlskrona.

Haargaard, B. and Fledelius, H.C. (2006) 'Down's syndrome and early cataract.' *British Journal of Ophthalmology 90*, 1024–1027.

Hall, G.R. (1994) 'Chronic dementia: Challenges in feeding the patient.' *Journal of Gerontologogical Nursing 15*, 16–20.

Hiatt, L.G. (1991) *Nursing Home Renovation Designed for Reform.* London: Butterworth Architecture.

Hiatt, L.G. (1995) 'Understanding the physical environment.' *Pride Institute Journal of Long Term Care 4*, 2 12–22.

Hofman, A., Rocco, W.A., Brayne, C., Breteler, M., Clarke, M. and Cooper, B. (1991) 'The prevalence of dementia in Europe: A collaborative study of 1980–1990 findings.' *International Journal of Epidemiology 20*, 736–748.

Holland, A.J. and Benton, M. (2004) *Ageing and its Consequences for People with Down's Syndrome: A Guide for Parents and Carers.* Teddington: Down's Syndrome Association.

Holland, A.J., Hon, J., Huppert, F.A. and Stevens, F. (2000) 'Incidence and course of dementia in people with Down's syndrome: Findings from a population-based study.' *Journal of Intellectual Disability Research 44*, 138–146.

Hopker, S. (1999) *Drug Treatments and Dementia – Bradford Dementia Group Good Practice Guide.* London: Jessica Kingsley Publishers.

Horgas, A. and Tsai, P. (1998) 'Analgesic drug prescription and use in cognitively impaired nursing homes residents.' *Nursing Research 47*, 4, 235.

Jacques, A. and Jackson, G. (2000) *Understanding Dementia* (3rd edition). Edinburgh: Churchill Livingstone.

Janicki. M. and Dalton, A. (eds) (1998) *Dementia, Aging and Intellectual Disabilities: A Handbook.* Philadelphia, PA: Brunner/Mazel.

Janicki, M. and Dalton, A. (2000) 'Prevalence of dementia and impact on intellectual disability services.' *Mental Retardation 38*, 3, 276–288.

Janicki, M., Davidson, P.W., Henderson, C.M., McCallion, P. *et al.* (2002) 'Health characteristics and health services utilization in older adults with intellectual disability.' *Journal of Intellectual Disability Research 46*, 4, 287–298.

Jenkins, D. (1998) *Bathing People with Dementia: The Bathroom and Beyond.* Stirling: Dementia Services Development Centre, University of Stirling.

Judd, S., Marshall, M. and Phippen, P. (1998) *Design for Dementia.* London: Hawker.

Julian, W. and Verriest, G. (1997) *Lighting Needs for the Partially Sighted.* Vienna: CIE Publications.

Kapell. D., Nightingale, B., Rodriguez, A., Lee, J.H., Zigman, W.B. and Schupf, N. (1998) 'Prevalence of chronic medical conditions in adults with mental retardation: Comparison with the general population.' *Mental Retardation 36*, 269–279.

Katzman, R. (1993) 'Education and the prevalence of dementia and Alzheimer's disease.' *Neurology 43*, 1, 13–20.

Kerr, D. (1997) *Down's Syndrome and Dementia: Practitioner's Guide.* Birmingham: Venture Press.

Kerr, D. and Cunningham, C. (2004) 'Finding the right response to people with dementia.' *Nursing and Residential Care 6*, 11, 539–542.

Kerr, D. and Innes, M. (2000) *What is Dementia? A Booklet for Adults with a Learning Disability.* Edinburgh: Scottish Down's Syndrome Association.

Kerr, D. and Wilkinson, H. (2005) *'In the Know': Implementing Good Practice: Information and Tools for Anyone Supporting People with a Learning Disability and Dementia.* Brighton: Pavilion.

Kerr, D. and Wilson, C. (eds) (2001) *Learning Disability and Dementia: A Training Guide for Staff.* Stirling: Dementia Services Development Centre, University of Stirling.

Kerr, D., Rae, C. and Wilkinson, H. (2002) '"Might it happen to me or not?" What do people with a learning disability understand about dementia?' *International Medical Review on Down's Syndrome 6*, 2, 27–30.

Kerr, D., Cunningham, C. and Wilkinson, H. (2006) *Responding to the Pain Needs of People with a Learning Disability and Dementia.* York: York Publishing Services.

Kiely, D.K., Morris, J.N., Algase, D.L. (2000) 'Resident characteristics associated with wandering in nursing homes.' *International Journal of Geriatric Psychiatry 15*, 1013–1020.

Killeen, J. (2000) *Planning Signpost for Dementia Care Services.* Edinburgh: Alzheimer Scotland Action on Dementia.

Kilstoff, K. and Chenoweth, L. (1998) 'New approaches to health and well being for dementia day care clients, family carers and day care staff.' *International Journal of Nursing Practice 4*, 1, 70–83.

Kitwood, T. (1997) *Dementia Reconsidered: The Person Comes First.* Milton Keynes: Open University Press.

Koncelik, J.A. (2003) 'The human factors of aging and the micro-environment: Personal surroundings, technology and product development.' *Journal of Housing for the Elderly 17*, 1, 117–134.

Kovach, C. and Henschel, H. (1996) 'Planning activities for patients with dementia: A descriptive study of therapeutic activities on special care units.' *Journal of Gerontological Nursing 22*, 9, 33–38.

Lai, F, and Williams, R.S. (1989) 'A prospective study of Alzheimer disease in Down's syndrome.' *Archives of Neurology 46*, 849•853.

Lennox, N. and Eastgate, G. (2004) 'Adults with intellectual disability and the GP.' *Australian Family Physician 33*, 8, 601–606.

Lewis, N. (2003) 'A life well lived.' *Down'ss Syndrome Association Journal 102.*

Livingston, S. (2003) 'Effective interventions to support medicine use in older people.' *Pharmaceutical Journal 270*, 893–895.

Lund, J. (1985) 'The prevalence of psychiatric morbidity in mentally retarded adults.' *Acta Psychiatrica Scandinavica 72*, 563–570.

Lynch, M.W., Rutecki, P.A. and Sutula, T.P. (1996) 'The effects of seizures on the brain.' *Current Opinion in Neurology 9*, 97–102.

McCaffery, M.S. (1968) *Nursing Theories Related to Cognition, Bodily Pain, and Man-Environment Interactions.* Los Angeles: UCLA Students Store.

McClean, W. (2000) *Practise Guide for Pain Management for People with Dementia in Institutional Care.* Stirling: Dementia Services Development Centre, University of Stirling.

McClean, W. (2003) 'Pain in clients with dementia: advocacy, ethics and treatment'. *Nursing and Residential Care* 5, 10, 482.

McGrother, C., Thorp, C., Taub, N. and Machado, O. (2001) 'Prevalence, disability and need in adults with severe learning disability.' *Tizard Learning Disability Review 6*, 4–13.

McKeith, I.G., Galasko, D., Wilcock, G.K. and Byrne, E.J. (1995) 'Lewy body dementia: Diagnosis and treatment.' *British Journal of Psychiatry 1167*, 6, 709–717.

McShane, R., Gedling, K., Kenward, B., Kenward, R., Hope, T. and Jacoby, R. (1998) 'The feasibility of electronic tracking devices in dementia: A telephone survey and case series.' *International Journal of Geriatric Psychiatry 13*, 556–563.

Malone, L. (1996) *Mealtimes and Dementia.* Stirling: Dementia Services Development Centre, University of Stirling.

Mani, C. (1988) 'Hypothyroidism in Down's syndrome.' *British Journal of Psychiatry 153*, 102–105.

Mason, J. and Scior, K. (2004) '"Diagnostic overshadowing" amongst clinicians working with people with intellectual disabilities in the UK.' *Journal of Intellectual Disability Research 47*, 1, 16–25.

Matson, J. (1982) 'The treatment of behavioural characteristics in the mentally retarded.' *Behaviour Therapy 13*, 209–218.

Meisen, B. (1993) 'Alzheimer's disease, the phenomenon of parent fixation and Bowlby's attachment theory.' *International Journal of Geriatric Psychiatry 8*, 147–153.

Mencap (2006) www.mencap.org.uk/html/about_learning_disability/learning_disability_conditions.asp (Accessed 4 January 2007).

Meyer, L.H. and Evans, I.M. (1994) *Nonaversive Interventions for Behavioural Problems.* Baltimore, MD: Paul H Brookes.

Michau, P. (1996) *Safety Call and Localisation of Elderly and Disabled People (SCALP) State of the Art Review and User Requirements Specification.* C/o Human Sciences and Advanced Technology Institute, Loughborough University.

Miller, E. and Morris, R. (1993) *The Psychology of Dementia.* Chichester: John Wiley.

Miskelly, F. (2004) 'A novel system of electronic tagging in patients with dementia and wandering.' *Age and Ageing 33*, 304–306.

Molloy, D.M. and Lubinksi, R. (1995) 'Dementia: Impact and Clinical Perspectives.' In R. Lubinski (ed.) *Dementia and Communication.* San Diego, CA: Singular.

Moniz-Cook, E., Woods, R., Gardener, E. (2000) 'Staff factors associated with perceptions of behaviour as "challenging" in residential and nursing homes.' *Aging Mental Health 4*, 1, 48–55.

Moss, S. and Patel, P. (1993) 'The prevalence of mental illness in people with intellectual disability over 50 years of age and the diagnostic importance of information from carers.' *Irish Journal of Psychology 14*, 110–129.

Murphy, C. (1994) *'It started with a Sea-shell': Life Story Work and People with Dementia.* Stirling: Dementia Services Development Centre, University of Stirling.

Naidu, R.S., Pratelli, P., Robinson, P.G. and Gelbier, S. (2001) 'The oral health and treatment needs of adults with a learning disability living in private households in Lambeth, Southwark and Lewisham, London.' *Journal of Disability and Oral Health 2*, 2, 78–82.

National Institute for Health and Clinical Excellence (NICE) (2006) *Dementia: Supporting People with Dementia and their Carers in Health and Social Care.* London: NICE.

Ng, J. and Li, S. (2003) 'A survey exploring the educational needs of care practitioners in learning disability in relation to death, dying and people with learning disabilities.' *European Journal of Cancer Care 12*, 12–19.

NHS Health Scotland (2004) *Health Needs Assessment Report: People with Learning Disabilities in Scotland.* Glasgow: Health Scotland.

Nor, K., McIntosh, I.B., Jackson, G.A. (2005) *Vascular Dementia: Series for Clinicians.* Stirling: Dementia Services Development Centre, University of Stirling.

O'Brien, J. (1987) 'A Guide to Life-Style Planning: Using *The Activities Catalog* to Integrate Services and Natural Support Systems.' In B. Wilcox and G.T. Bellamy (eds) *A Comprehensive Guide to the Activities Catalog: An Alternative Curriculum for Youth and Adults with Severe Disabilities.* Baltimore, MD: Paul H. Brookes.

O'Leary, E. and Barry, N. (1998) 'Reminiscence therapy with older adults.' *Journal of Social Work Practice 12*, 2, 159–165.

Oliver, C. (1998) 'Perspectives on Assessment and Evaluation.' In M. Janicki and A. Dalton (eds) *Dementia, Aging and Intellectual Disabilities: A Handbook.* Philadelphia, PA: Brunner/Mazel.

Osborn, C. (1999) *The Reminiscence Handbook: Ideas for Creative Activities with Older People.* London: Age Exchange.

Oswin, M. (1991) 'Am I Allowed to Cry?' A Study of Bereavement amongst People who have Learning Difficulties. London: Souvenir Press.

Pollock, A. (2001) Designing Gardens for People with Dementia. Stirling: Dementia Service Development Centre, University of Stirling.

Pollock, R. (2007) Lighting and People with Dementia. Stirling: Dementia Services Development Centre, University of Stirling.

Prasher, V.P (1995) 'Age-specific prevalence: Thyroid dysfunction and depressive symptomology in adults with Down's syndrome and dementia.' International Journal of Geriatric Psychiatry 10, 25–31.

Prasher, V.P. (1999) 'Down's syndrome and thyroid disorders: A review.' Down's Syndrome Research and Practice 6, 25–42.

Prasher, V.P. (2005) Alzheimer's Disease and Dementia in Down's Syndrome and Intellectual Disabilities. Oxford: Radcliffe.

Prasher, V.P. and Krishnan, V.H.R. (1993) 'Age of onset and duration of dementia in people with Down's syndrome: Integration of 98 reported cases in the literature.' International Journal of Geriatric Psychiatry 8, 915–922.

Prasher, V.P., Cumella, S., Natarajan, K., Rolfe, R., Shah, S. and Haque, M.S. (2003) 'Magnetic resonance imaging, Down's syndrome and Alzheimer's disease: Research and clinical implications.' Journal of Intellectual Disability Research 47, 2, 90–100.

Prinsley, D.M. (1986) 'Music therapy in geriatric care.' Australian Nurses Journal 15, 9, 22–26.

Puyenbroeck, J. and Maes, B. (2002) 'Reminiscence in older people with learning disabilities: An exploratory study.' Paper presented at the Inaugural Conference of the International Association for the Scientific Study of Intellectual Disability-Europe, Dublin, 12–15 June.

Ragnoskog, H. (1994) 'Dinner, Music and Dementia.' In Towards the Third Millennium Conference Proceedings. Adelaide: Flinders Nurses Education and Research Funding, quoted in J. Granville-Short Counselling Strategies, MindaInc Volume 2. Brighton, South Australia.

Rainbow, A. (2003) The Reminiscence Skills Training Book. Bicester: Speechmark.

Robertson, J., Emerson, E., Gregory, N., Hatton, C., Kessissoglou, S. and Hallam, A. (2000) 'Receipt of psychotropic medication by people with learning disability in residential settings.' Journal of Intellectual Disability Research 44, 6, 666–676.

Ryden, M., Bossenmaier, M. and McLauchlan, C. (1991) 'Aggressive behaviour in cognitively impaired nursing home residents.' Research in Nursing and Health 14, 87–95.

Sander, R. (2002) 'Standing and moving: Helping people with vascular dementia.' Nursing Older People 14, 1, 20–26.

Scottish Executive (2000) The Same as You: A Review of Services for People with Learning Disabilities. Edinburgh: The Stationery Office.

Scottish Intercollegiate Guidelines Network (SIGN) (1986) Management of Patients with Dementia. A National Guideline. Edinburgh: Scottish Intercollegiate Guidelines Network.

Selby, P. (2001) Diabetes and Down's Syndrome: Notes for Parents and Carers. London: Down's Syndrome Association.

Stokes, G. and Goudie, F. (1990) Working with Dementia. Bicester: Winslow Press.

Stuart-Hamilton, I. (2000) The Psychology of Ageing: An Introduction (3rd edition). London: Jessica Kingsley Publishers.

Surrey and Borders Partnership NHS Trust (2006) Eating and Drinking Safely: A Concern for Us All. A Joint Surrey and Borders Partnership NHS Trust, Speech and Language Therapist and Dietetic Project: 18 Mole Business Park, Leatherhead, Surrey, KT22 7AD.

Taylor, F. (2006) 'Positive applications of assistive technology in the community.' Journal of Dementia Care 14, 5, 9.

Teri, L. and Logsdon, R.G. (1991) 'Identifying pleasant activities for Alzheimer's disease patients: The pleasant events schedule-AD.' The Gerontologist 31, 1, 124–127.

Thompson, D. and Wright, S. (2001) Misplaced and Forgotten: People with Learning Disabilities in Residential Services for Older People. London: Mental Health Foundation.

Tsai, P. and Chang, J. (2004) 'Assessment of pain in elders with dementia'. Medsurg Nursing 13, 6, 364–90.

Utton, D. (2007) Designing Homes for People with Dementia. London: Journal of Dementia Care and Hawker Publications.

Van Schrojenstein Lantman-De Valk, H.M.J., Metsemakers, J.F.M., Havenman, M.J. and Crebolder, H.F.J.M. (2000) 'Health problems in people with intellectual disability in general practice: A comparative study.' Family Practice 17, 5, 405–407.

VOICES (Voluntary Organisations Involved in Caring in the Elderly Sector) (1998) *Eating Well for Older People with Dementia: A Good Practice Guide for Residential and Nursing Homes and Others Involved in Caring for Older People with Dementia: Report of an Expert Working Group.* Potters Bar: VOICES and Gardner Merchant Healthcare Services.

Watson, R. (1994) 'Measuring feeding difficulty in patients with dementia: Replication and validation of the EdFED scale 1.' *Journal of Advanced Nursing 19,* 850–855.

Wey, S. (2006) '"Working in the Zone": A Social-ecological Framework for Dementia Rehabilitation.' In J. Woolham (ed.) *Assistive Technology in Dementia Care.* London: Hawker.

Wherret, J.R. (1998) 'Neurological Aspects.' In M.P. Janicki and A.J. Dalton (eds) *Dementia, Aging and Intellectual Disabilities: A Handbook.* Philadelphia, PA: Brunner/Mazel.

Wilkinson, H., Kerr, D. and Rae C. (2003) 'People with a learning disability: Their concerns about dementia.' *Journal of Dementia Care 11,* 27–29.

Wilkinson, H., Kerr, D., Cunningham, C. and Rae, C. (2004) *'Home for Good?' Models of Good Practice for Supporting People with a Learning Disability and Dementia.* Brighton: Pavilion.

Wilkinson, H., Kerr, D. and Cunningham, C. (2005) 'Equipping staff to support people with an intellectual disability and dementia in care home settings.' *Dementia: International Journal of Social Research 4,* 3, 387–400.

Wolfensberger, W. (1972) *Normalisation: The Principles of Normalisation in Human Services.* Toronto: National Institute on Mental Retardation.

Woods, B., Spector, A., Jones, C., Orrell, M. and Davies, S. (2006) 'Reminiscence therapy for dementia.' *Cochrane Database of Systematic Reviews* (CD001120).

World Health Organization (WHO) (1992) *International Classification of Diseases and Related Health Problems – Tenth Revision* (ICD 10). Geneva: WHO.

World Health Organization (WHO) (1996) *Cancer Pain Relief: With a Guide to Opioid Availability* (2nd edition). Geneva: WHO.

Wright, D., Chapman, N., Foundling-Miah, M., Greenwall, R. *et al.* (2006) *Consensus Guideline on the Medication Management of Adults with Swallowing Difficulties.* Bristol: Connect Medical.

Subject Index

Author Index

1928